Resilient Aging AND Wellness

MINDFUL STEWARDSHIP
OF BODY, MIND, AND SPIRIT
INTO THE NEXT SEASON OF LIVING

Resilient Aging is a must read for Baby Boomers, Gen Xr's, Millennials and/or just about anyone with a desire to peer into your future and create and build a positive image and a future healthy life. Physical and/or cognitive frailty are not ubiquitous but occur way too often in our present generation of older adults. You now have an opportunity to open up the door with keys to success in the adoption of healthy lifestyle behaviors and the screening and managing common age-related diseases, all while enhancing your spiritual and psychological inner self. Dr. Eckrich has carefully crafted a number of chapters that will keep you up to date on the latest way to honor your temple (your body) and your mind. A must read!

David B. Carr, MD
Washington University School of Medicine
Alan A. and Edith L. Wolff Professor of Geriatric Medicine
Professor of Medicine and Neurology
Clinical Director
Division of Geriatrics and Nutritional Science

As I get older, I notice changes in my body, in my thinking, in my disposition. As I change, I sometimes experience excitement and anticipation, but as of late I more often become unsettled and sometimes apprehensive. As a physician and as a believer in Jesus Christ, Dr. Eckrich explores the ways I am aging based on his years of the medical care of others and his experience as a devout reader of Scripture. This book explains my experiences of growing older from the perspectives of both the physician's eyes and the eyes of faith. This is a perceptive and insightful guide and reference work for caregivers and for care receivers and especially for us who are not getting any younger.

Rev. Dr. Robert Kolb
Professor of Systematic Theology, Concordia Seminary, Saint Louis, MO

As the president of a leading senior living housing and services provider in the United States, I was captivated by the way that Dr. Eckrich connected all the dots in the aging process. He helps readers understand how the way they live impacts the aging process physically, mentally, and spiritually. This book provides a nice balance of practical medical advice with a strong connection to spiritual values. This information can not only prolong your life but also improve your quality of life in the aging process.

John Kotovsky
President and CEO
Lutheran Senior Services

We're living longer and how! Can't argue with the *how* of these substantive, well-documented aging facts. We can ignore them, but they'll remind us in the morning! Dr. Eckrich teaches *how* our aches and pains are countered with gains. He prescribes a perspective to adapt downturns of mind, body, and soul into *bouncebackability!* These pages ponder "pause and pivot of the soul," as well as the abs that are in and tightening the skin! Such optimism springs from decades as an internist, facing life and death issues with patients, and from personal experience. His contagious hope is founded on the proven track record of the Creator of Life whose gift of resiliency is yours for the asking. You were made for such a time, such an age as this! Turn the page and dive in to "older but wiser!" Or as Eckrich puts it, "into overcoming the gene pool" even if we're swimming upstream!

Phyllis Wallace
Host, Syndicated Christian Women's Talk Show "Woman to Woman"
Speaker, Author

Dr. Eckrich takes us on a resilient journey through the aging process by sharing his experiences and knowledge as a person of God, medical doctor, family man, and trainer of others. He shows us how we can celebrate God's gift of aging every day! The book brings a fresh meaning to the word "resilient" by emphasizing how we can adapt to the various changes and life tasks that we all face in positive and creative ways. This is not a textbook of medical terms and research but rather a gift for the reader to use to navigate through a life of wellness and, yes, of course, resilience. Here's to "resilient aging" in the Lord!"

Dr. Rich Bimler
Ambassador of Health, Hope, and Aging (AH-HA!)
Ministry Consultant

The aging process can be depressing and distressing, or it can be full of new experiences and new ways of serving God. This is the refreshing insight of Dr. Eckrich who, as a medical doctor and also a student of the Bible, puts together a map of "resilient aging." Through this excellent book, he gives insight into how the Christian can remain responsive to changing environments throughout the aging process. Key to his thinking is the necessity of the soul to remain connected to Christ. This fundamental identity is the "set point" in the homeostatic systems of the soul that leads to resilient aging. His Bible quotation says it all: "So we do not lose heart. Though outwardly we are wasting away yet inwardly we are being renewed day by day." (2 Corinthians 4:16) The key is living a life of purpose, a life of movement, a life of nutritious eating, and a life with good relationships in community and family. There is no retirement as a Christian, only repositioning to continue to serve God well!

Rev. Dr. David Ludwig
Clergyman and Professor of Psychology
Lenore Rhyne University, Hickory, NC

There are two requisites for wellness: one physical, the other spiritual. We can readily understand how a physician of many years can speak to the physical. But Dr. Eckrich speaks with authority to the spiritual as well. And he doesn't simply leave it as an encouragement to invite the Creator into our lives. He gives compelling evidence as to how that relationship improves our lives as we make our way into the next season of life and eternity. Dr. Eckrich emboldens us not only to conquer life, but also to conquer death in Christ as well. Oh, yes, and he touches on how to "do" retirement well too. He pretty much covers the essentials for aging resiliently!

Ty Dodge
Chairman Emeritus, Realty South
Elder, Briarwood Presbyterian Church (PCA)
Lay counselor, Bible teacher

This book reads like the owner's manual for a full, healthy, resilient life! Beginning with the Creator's plan for full, healthy, and perfect life, Dr. Eckrich takes us past the Fall into sin and into the life we can choose while we are still on this side of heaven where full health will be restored. Dr. Eckrich points out that the way to actually *thrive* is to have a vibrant faith life, healthy relationships, wise physical choices—and it doesn't hurt to eat foods that are good for you! You'll return to this helpful, practical book again and again to understand how the human body ages, what you can do in the midst of those changes, and the secrets of resiliency. Dr. Eckrich faithfully affirms that we are fearfully and wonderfully made.

Ruth Koch, MA, NCC
Mental Health Educator
Women's and Family's Issues Author and Lecturer

Aging is a given. Resilient aging is not. Dr. Eckrich shines light on the path to live our last decades with health and grace.

Rev. Dr. Robert DeWetter
Senior Pastor Snowmass Chapel
Episcopal Priest and Clinical Psychologist

All of us grow old; this is simply an inescapable fact of life. For most of us, this realization starts to hit in our forties when things previously done effortlessly are no longer so effortless. Dr. Eckrich guides the reader on a practical and thoughtful path to discover how critical resiliency is in our later years. The topic of resiliency is all the rage in psychology, psychiatry, and the behavioral sciences; however, this book is unique. In addition to discussing the physical nature of resiliency, Dr. Eckrich also addresses the emotional and spiritual aspects from a Christian theological perspective, emphasizing that resiliency is quintessentially tied into our connection with God. It is a thoughtful and thought-provoking book that supplies practical and spiritual help in developing resilience in the "next season."

Charles R. Conway, MD
Professor of Psychiatry
Washington University School of Medicine
Director, Washington University Treatment-Resistant Depression Clinic

Resilient Aging and Wellness

MINDFUL STEWARDSHIP
OF BODY, MIND, AND SPIRIT
INTO THE NEXT SEASON OF LIVING

JOHN D. ECKRICH, M.D.

TENTH
POWER

Elgin, IL · Tyler, TX

TENTHPOWERPUBLISHING
www.tenthpowerpublishing.com

Design by Inkwell Creative.

Softcover 978-1-938840-17-3

e-book 978-1-938840-18-0

10 9 8 7 6 5 4 3 2 1

To those who strive to bequeath genes, jeans, genius,
and Jesus to the next generation

TABLE OF CONTENTS

ACKNOWLEDGEMENTS

The breadth of topics covered in *Resilient Aging and Wellness* are served well by the collaborators who have reviewed and edited sections of this text.

I offer thanks to physicians at Washington University School of Medicine in St. Louis who specialize in geriatrics and cognitive function, especially Dr. David Carr, Professor of Geriatrics and Internal Medicine and Director of the Rehabilitation Center at Washington University, for his insight into both the process and changes of physical and cognitive aging, but also therapies to add resilience. I would also like to thank Dr. Charles Conway, Professor of Psychiatry at Washington University School of Medicine for his review and guidance of cognitive care in aging. I greatly appreciate the assistance of Stephanie Paule, MS, Fellowship Program Coordinator, Division of Geriatrics and Nutritional Science at Washington University School of Medicine for her research of the literature regarding physical and cognitive aging in contemporary science and medicine.

I would also like to recognize Craig Schnuck, Chairman Emeritus of Schnuck Markets, Inc. in St. Louis and Chairman of the board of directors of Washington University in St. Louis. His connections and guidance to outstanding resources of that medical faculty have been invaluable.

Two professors of theology at Concordia Seminary, St. Louis, have added greatly to the understanding of the spirit and soul provided in the Holy Scriptures and the practical application of God's Word to the difficult questions we raise regarding beginning, continuance, and end of life mysteries that all of us face as we age. Rev. Dr. Robert Kolb, Professor Emeritus of Systematic Theology, and Rev. Dr. Jeffrey Gibbs, Professor of Exegetical Theology, have shared their time and learned wisdom to enlighten this discussion.

I wish to thank Jim Dankenbring, Esq., attorney and partner at Spencer Fane, LLP, for his review and suggestions regarding end of life estate planning and legal documentation. In this same subject, I am also thankful to David Hoffman, Chairman Emeritus of USI insurance services for reviewing later life health insurance care considerations.

I appreciate the encouragement and partnership of Rev. Dr. Robert DeWetter, Senior Pastor of Snowmass Chapel, Snowmass, Colorado and licensed clinical psychologist, as well as Pastor Charla Belinski, Associate Pastor of Snowmass Chapel as we have jointly shared precursors of this material in seminars in Aspen Valley. Also, I appreciate the insight provided by our personal pastor, Rev. Dr. Scott Seidler, Senior Pastor of Concordia Lutheran Church, Kirkwood, Missouri, whose sermons on spiritual care have been insightful and inspiring.

I wish to express much appreciation to Mark Zimmermann for his masterful editing guidance, particularly on the topic of spirituality in aging.

As always, we have a wonderful staff at Grace Place Wellness Ministries based in St. Louis, who have kindly reviewed this material for grammatical accuracy and content. This staff includes Randy Fauser, President and CEO; Rev. Dr. Darrell Zimmerman, VP of Programming; Beth McAnallen, Retreat Coordinator; and Kathy Greffet, Office Manager. Thanks, team!

As with my previous books, I wish to acknowledge the team at Tenth Power Publishing for their highly professional and meticulous guidance in the process of bringing this to life, including Jim and Kathe Galvin, Mary Ann Lackland, and artist Lindsay Ann Taylor.

Finally, I wish to thank my dear wife Kathy for her patience and support and my children Chris, Molly, and Barclay, and Michael and Annie and first grandchild Greyson for their encouragement and understanding.

At the last, I thank the many patients, colleagues, and friends from more than 45 years of medical practice for all the perspectives on aging well that have formed the foundation of this book. I thank and praise the Lord for his steadfast love given to me and to us all that gives us hope through the healing of the Cross and the power of the Resurrection.

Deo Gloria

INTRODUCTION

Okay, have you ever taken a few moments to pause and ponder what this whole *aging process* is all about? If you picked up this book, I'm guessing you have. Here's a chance to take both a "pause point" and potentially a "pivot point" with a physician at your side who is aging right along with you. I invite you to read, reflect, and creatively *reform* your understanding of *where you are* and *how you might proceed* with your journey into the next season of life. I am encouraging you to be *mindful* (aware of what's important) as you make choices to care for and steward your health and vitality as you age. You can't stop getting older, but you can significantly influence the ways in which you respond to the changes occurring within your being—you can affect *how* you age.

I hope you will compare *how* you *are* in reference to your fellow aging travelers, particularly in light of the wealth of scientific, cultural, and spiritual *wellbeing* conversation churning about in the 21st century. Determining your comparative-wellness status is not to inflate or depress your self-worth or sense of relative wellbeing. Rather, it is to better understand the challenges and choices each of us face daily as constantly changing persons, so that we might remain functional and joyful for as long as we are able. Additionally, it is just as critical that we learn from and encourage each other. There appears to be great value in being mutually accountable as we age.

I'm asking you to consider how you fit in with the whole of your generation and how you are influencing the next generations by your choices, your lifestyle, and your legacy of health behavior. Consequentially, I am asking you to think about what's *next* for you, me, and our fellow aging colleagues—and if what's next *is* in any way under our actual sphere of influence.

If you are like me, it seems a lot of what's changing in us as we age is beyond our control. Often, it feels as if we are riding on the crest of a sinister wave that is picking up intensity and speed of its own volition.

One significant factor producing that sense of powerless apprehension is the reality of losing *resiliency* with aging—losing the capacity to *spring* back or to return to a healthy baseline. It feels like our body, in its whole and in its parts, lessens its ability to achieve *homeostasis* (stable equilibrium). Our organs and systems can't return to a *set-point* as readily to face the next series of stresses and strains as they did years ago. I will examine these concepts of biological, psychological, and spiritual *resilience, homeostasis,* and *set-points* in depth as we journey through this text together.

The study of the biological, social, cultural, psychological, and cognitive aspects of aging is called *gerontology. Gerontologists* reveal that nearly 80% of the determinants for the length and quality of life for 21st-century earthlings may be due to how we move, eat, and interact rather than merely due to a set of passed-down parental and grandparental genes. Genes are important, to be sure; but how they fulfill their *blueprint* for our lives often is determined by other extra-genetic influences. Having said that *nurture* (life style) might have a stronger influence on lifespan and life-quality than *nature* (genetics), I have yet to see a set of genes living apart from its environment.

An additional longevity and wellbeing enhancement factor appears to be our desire and ability to *downshift,* to deploy to a quieter and slower pace of living regularly or at least intermittently throughout our day. Physically and mentally *resting* routinely seems to restore resilience to both the human creature and all of creation.

Furthermore, many of us are reasonably healthy, vibrant, cognizant, and financially able to leave the life-tasks and professions that carried us into our late fifties and sixties, and are now considering what we might do *next.* That may not have always been the historical context of our ancestors.

Stereotypical retirement activities like golf, bridge, grandparenting, or volunteering, while all enjoyable and much appreciated, may not be satisfying enough to consume all of our time and energy.

I'm guessing in many ways the discussion I'm about to share with you will ring pleasant or onerous chimes within your life as a *Boomer, Gen X-er, or Millennial*. I suspect your family, hometown, education, career or vocation, and opportunities might differ from mine. Yet, to provide at least one post-WWII example, here's a capsular look at—well—me. I've had the opportunity to lead the joyful, as well as stressful and challenging life of a physician. I suspect that your careers as lawyers, teachers, farmers, pastors, businesspersons, IT managers, maintenance persons, home/family managers, or numerous other callings were equally fulfilling. Additionally, I do know this: you too were extensively challenged; not always rewarded as you thought deserving of your efforts; most likely disrespected as often as praised; and you too experienced substantial stress on a daily basis.

At age 60, I *changed* careers. At age 70, I'm *changing* directions again. This may be similar to your work history at various life-crossroads. Or you may have worked at Bendix for 40 years and received the gold watch, although that is not the career path of most Americans these days.[1] Medical and immunological science, personal choices, behavioral adjustments, fiscal stability, and—most importantly—God's good *grace* are making these directional shifts possible for me and might be for you. You'll note I neglect to list *luck* in my influencing factors. You may disagree and contribute what happens to you as *destiny*, or *chance*, or *the roll of the dice*. That is not my view. I believe we are blessed by God with a free will and choices; we each experience confrontations and opportunities. Are you ready to deal effectively with the change that inherently accompanies choice, challenges, and aging?

As a physician who also is a Christian, I believe there is something much more powerful and significant than *serendipity* at work here. This unique entity we identify as *human*—this *body-mind-spirit* creature unique in the earth and the heavens—this *relational being* breathed to life by a relational Creator and restored to God's family by God's relational Son—I believe has purpose and mission. We are not random chance. If you think we are, you may be troubled by the direction of this thought piece.

Therefore, the relevant journey behind, at hand, and before us holds meaning and purpose for us, our neighbor, and our Creator. And I firmly believe that as humans, we have been granted a will which leads to the ability to choose from divergent paths in the *yellow wood* of our life.[2]

This is a remarkable season in the history of humankind. The hopeful task of this book is to help us understand what happens to our bodies, minds, and spirits in aging. Despite possessing aging material substance (i.e., hearts, brains, skin, gastrointestinal systems, etc.), older cognitive property (thought, perception, memory, emotions, etc.), and an active, ongoing relationship with our Creator, we have choice. I am convinced that we have newer and dynamic opportunities to pursue ever-creative visions and fulfilling-missions for living and serving God and God's people with joy and with abundance.

I invite and urge you to pursue *resilience* within the daily health and wellness decisions before you. Take care of yourself, not selfishly, but as a caretaker of the gift of life itself.

"Do you not know that your bodies are temples of the Holy Spirit, who is in you, whom you have received from God?" (1 Corinthians 6:19)

Another way to state this is that I hope this book provides insight into how you might *mindfully steward* your body, mind, spirit, relationships, and resources to add vitality, effectiveness, joyfulness, and meaning no matter where you find yourself on your life's course.

From our Christian faith perspective, we are assured that the fountain, the living water at the core of resilience, stewardship, and purpose, comes from the Cross, and its former inhabitant in our stead, God's Son, Jesus Christ. With such a gift and resource in hand, my prayer for you is knowledge, understanding of purpose, active living, meaningful legacy, and assurance of being loved and of loving, especially in your later years. And, let's make this wellness-walk *together*. Let's extend our hands to our fellow travelers wherever they might appreciate a little lift. I know I have been supported by many good and indispensable souls and I deeply appreciate their grips of friendship. I'll share one final, fundamental feature for meaningful aging: love.

Godspeed & God's grace!

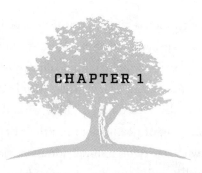

CHAPTER 1

AGING AS A HUMAN BEING

I t is a fact of life that we as humans age. From the moment we are born, we are growing older. As we reach into our later years, the effects of the aging of our bodies and our minds can be seen and felt more profoundly. But like with many circumstances in life, our focus should not be only about aging itself but our response to it. God has given us a unique ability to be *resilient* in aging and to find wellness in our later years. As a medical physician who is Christian, I have seen resilient aging and wellness at work in those I treated and I have witnessed the positive impact of a Christ-centered life on physical, cognitive, and spiritual health. Understanding and embracing aging from a Christian perspective is fundamental for us of Christian faith in experiencing a rich and fulfilling stage of older age. It is so because it encompasses into the activity of aging a recognition and inclusion of that which binds body and mind together—that binding agent or *religio* in Latin—our spirituality, our relationship to our Creator.

As you may have noticed, there has been a surge in our society regarding our understanding of getting older. Specifically there is currently a revolution in the healthcare of aging. A recent headline in my local paper reads, "Aging in Aspen: How Long Do You Want To Live?" The article reviews the work of J. Craig Venter, an early pioneer in the quest to sequence the human genome, and his new venture called Human Longevity, Inc., headquartered in La Jolla, California.[3]

Human Longevity, Inc., is aimed at providing people with the most complete and intensive genetic and physical assessment of their health that has ever been available. These are literally "roadmaps" showing subscribers to this service, in intimate detail, exactly where their bodies are in the aging process. The service identifies through DNA what disorders, including cancer, exist within them or potentially lie in their future, based on their genetics coupled with powerful, non-radiation emitting, full-body MRI scans. The potential benefit is to give people advanced information on preexisting health risks so that aggressive preventive healthcare can be initiated at an early point in life.

While this type of approach can have worth, the truth is that it still cannot foresee all of the many other variables that affect our heath as we age. That is why currently, we more often use the longstanding traditional approach to aging, which is to treat problems once they are established and evident. You and your doctor can also assess the role of the fuel you feed yourself, the toxins you might be exposed to, the amount of exercise and movement you afford yourself, and the availability of family and friends to surround and support you. In addition, you and your physician must wrestle with whether or not the benefits are greater than the risks for certain treatments. You and your medical care team must determine which wellness *prescriptions* will add not just longevity but also quality to your life.

The most positive impact I have seen in my 45 years as a primary care physician on the process of aging is a healthy mind and spirit in concert with a healthy body. As people of faith, we understand that our bodies decline because of sin; eventually, our bodies cease to function completely—we die. Along the way, many if not most of us will also encounter a faltering mind—ours. However, as people of faith, we understand that we are gifted with a *new life in Christ*. Christ renews our beings every day in his love, forgiveness, and salvation. As St. Paul writes, "Therefore we do not lose heart. Though outwardly we are wasting away, yet inwardly we are being renewed day by day." (2 Corinthians 4:16)

I return to the reality of life as a human that we *all* age, and I hope I'm not the first one to let you know this—you'll find out in due time. We humans are mortal creatures. As we age, there is natural *change* and a general *decline* in our human ability to deal with our internal and external environment; we lose *resilience* or the ability to *spring back*.

Do we have insight into what causes the decline in resiliency in humankind? *Scientists* might blame deteriorating energy fields, buildup of toxins, or damage due to DNA oxidation or DNA methylation within cells for the declining viability. Those are complex words and complicated concepts; nonetheless, we will take a peek at DNA maintenance and cell death later in the section on aging of our immune system. Furthermore, revelations are occurring almost daily around the newer work on the shortening of chromosomal end zones called *telomeres*.[4]

Sociologists, from their perspective, might point out that our culture is deteriorating so rapidly and family structure is so unstable that we are losing our ability to adapt.

However, as a scientist of Christian faith, I understand that these eventualities were not always the case and not the scenario of Adam and Eve as they were first created. Their sin and our sin usher in deterioration, suffering, and death. (Romans 6:23) Sin and the perpetual presence of our sinful behavior (living with a focus on self rather than our connection to God) are at the root of a fallen creation. But Christ came to reverse the curse of sin and make us new creations through his death on the cross and resurrection from the grave. Through Christ, we already know the outcome of our personal stories: we have everlasting life when our journey on this earth comes to an end.

Perhaps a more pertinent question for us, therefore, is: Can we age more *successfully* or remain *more responsive* to our changing environment as faithful Christians until death claims us? Can we more *meaningfully* occupy space on this planet by being able to continue to contribute in a Christ-like way? In other words, can we age more purposefully, joyfully, and functionally? I believe that question is the main question for us all.

I suggest to you that one definition of a *successful aging process* might be one that allows us to *respond and adjust appropriately and resiliently to the fundamentally diminishing capabilities of our human elements in relation to our altering circumstances and our Christian faith.*

Therefore, if we are aging successfully and resiliently, our BODIES— our organs, pump, and wiring giving us breath, heartbeat, and activity within each cell in our body, and the ability to protect ourselves from threats—remain responsive and coordinated. Our MINDS—alertness, sensible thoughts, perceptions, memory, and emotional responses—are clear, appropriate, and helpful. And our SPIRITS—a sharp and sure understanding of how we relate and interact with ourselves, others, and our Creator; our understanding of our identity, who and whose we are; and our desire and ability to fear, love, and trust as our Creator unconditionally loves us—are vibrant, peaceful, and focused outward to God and others rather than into ourselves.

I am sure each of us is aware of those dealing with diminished body function, limited cognition due to stroke, dementia, or depression, or struggling in their spiritual life, perhaps within our own families. Our society might suggest a lessening of their considered human value or ability to contribute to the wellbeing of our tribe. However, this is not their *meaning* or *worth* in God's eyes, nor should it be in ours. What an opportunity, what an invitation, what a privilege it is for us to extend our helping and encouraging hands into the journeys of those struggling so as to clothe them, feed them, shelter them, assure them justice, and share with them God's Word. We can purposefully pursue resilience with them.

Inescapably, the linking of arms to the most challenged of our society brings enormous richness into the lives of all in the human family.

So why strive for resiliency? I think it is a matter of personal *stewardship*, not personal *meaning* or *worth*. Our Creator has given us the gift of a miraculous body, mind, and spirit; and yet, our whole being remains in a constant state of tension with sin. God's Word tells us that God expects us to be taking care of these most precious gifts wisely and mindfully, rather than neglecting or *burying* them in the earth. (Luke 16-1-13; 1 Peter 4:10) Our physical, cognitive, and spiritual beings are just as much a gift of God as any talent or resource.

As a physician of Christian conviction, therefore, my prescription for mindful aging that I am suggesting for you goes like this: to age well as a human requires that we age in a fashion that mindfully stewards (cares for) the gift of resilience in body, mind, and spirit, and their interactivity with each other, but is always founded, secure, and flowing from our relationship with our loving Creator. Our worth and wellness is all and all in Christ.

What Does It Mean to Be Human?

Several major dilemmas arise as we wrestle with a *prescription* to assist us in *resilient aging*, considering the plethora of variables and constants we face as humans.

The first major conundrum to consider is what does it mean to be *wholly human*? When we explore what happens to us as we age, and what we might do to maintain effective function and joyfulness of living, it is important to understand what it means to be a human in the first place.

For that we go to Rene Descartes (1596-1650), a Jesuit-trained French philosopher, mathematician, and scientist. Descartes searched for a way, from the perspective of a person of faith, to understand the new findings of science within the framework and teaching of the Holy Scriptures and the Church's traditional teachings. After a time, Descartes came to espouse *dualism* as a way to understand a human: humankind is made up of a physical body and a mind/soul. In his approach, the mind/soul controls the body, but the body also influences the mind/soul in a two-way interaction. The mind/soul-body relationship not only continues prominently in science and philosophy today, but Descartes' approach to breaking down component parts of the human being so that they can be studied, understood, and treated dominates much of medical science into the 21st century. (If you are interested in thoughts on humanness prior to Descartes, please see the appendix under *Historical Perspectives on Being Human*.)

Most interestingly, however, it is worth noting that Descartes boldly maintains the traditional religious idea of all in this world being created and dependent on God for its existence.[5]

Humanness in Contemporary Christian Thought: Capacity to Fear, Love, Trust

So let me now apply a 21st century *Christian* lens to this topic of *humanness*. In the early history of the Christian faith community, theologians as well as physicians, appear to struggle with what "makes up" a human being: dichotomists (body-soul) and trichotomists (spirit/soul-mind-body) abound in thought and writing. A leading Christian theologian of today, Rev. Dr. Robert Kolb, Emeritus Professor of Systematic Theology at Concordia Seminary, St. Louis, finds it more helpful, and more Biblical, to frame a contemporary discussion on humanness through considering the nature of being human as follows:

- We have a physical nature.

- We have a psychological/cognitive/emotional/volitional nature.

- We have a relational nature of the whole person to our Creator.

Some in traditional and contemporary Christian theological thought call part two the *soul*, and part three the *spirit*; yet others reverse the terminology. Whichever terms you utilize, our physical and cognitive components may change as we age, but the third component—our relationship with God—Dr. Kolb affirms, does not change because it is *dependent* on God; God's promise remains steady and sure. Our Creator is unchangeable and eternal. We, as humans, are not. However, our human perception of our relationship with God may, in fact, wax and wane.

Expanding 21st-century thought further, Dr. Teresa Iglesias, medical bioethicist and lecturer at Trinity International University, Dublin, and the University of Chicago, invites us to "pay attention" to three further fundamental aspects of being human:

- A human has a body, is organic, and is physical.

- A human is an integrated-unity-of-life, a whole entity from the beginning, and simultaneously an individual.

- The human is a being with a temporal continuity, a being with a history, a being in time.

The third bullet point is valuable to this discourse. We are not machines built by installments; we are formed or initiated at conception, potentiated with the genetic blueprints to grow, to think, to respond to whatever the environment presents to us—we are resilient. We are part of a process, but all our constituent parts are fully present from the beginning. We are also unified from the beginning, an organic whole. We grow as a whole, we interact with others as a whole, and we die as a whole.[6]

Non-human animals have bodies and animals have abilities to perceive, think, remember, and respond. Although there is substantial controversy, even in some Christian quarters, as to whether animals have souls, the Scriptures describe humankind as a particularly unique and blessed creature breathed into with the breath of God, made whole in God's image, and gifted to be a soul. (See the appendix under *Is the Soul Uniquely Human?*.)

So if we are a whole being (we are a soul and not just have a soul), the question becomes: What is *unique* in the nature of being human about the possession of a relationship with our Creator that is different from merely having a physical or a thinking nature? I believe framing our relationship with an unchanging, faithful, continuously engaged Creator, affords us the contemporaneous *capacity to fear, love, and trust that Creator.*

Love:

We might distill this *uniqueness* further by saying that the *image* of God breathed into man is *love*! We know God is by nature a relational God. In our Christian faith, God's Son, Jesus, flows from the Father through love. The Holy Spirit flows from the Father and the Son through love. God breathes into the creature we call human God's own image, the capacity to love and to be in love-filled relationships. Love gives us the ability to live *outwardly* in relationship with our Creator and with the rest of God's creation through that love, rather than an *inward* focus on self.[7]

Christian theologians from St. Ambrose and St. Augustine, through Martin Luther, and onto the 20th century's Frederick Bonhoeffer, define sin as turning inward to self *or incurvatus in se* (Latin). (See appendix.) In Christ's death and resurrection, we are created anew to live with our energy and focus in life flowing *outward* toward our Creator rather than *inward*. We are invited and empowered by Christ to fear, love, and trust in being a *New Creation.* (2 Corinthians 5:17) However, we understand that in our earthly walk we remain imperfect; we are sinful by our very nature and desires.

This uniqueness extends to our individuality; we were each created with different talents (Psalm 139:13-14; Isaiah 64:8); different purposes (Ephesians 2:10); different callings within the world and the Body of Christ (1 Corinthians 12:25-28); different spiritual gifts (1 Peter 4:10-11).

Fear and Trust:

That's a bit about love. What about *fear* and *trust*? The Scriptures provide us with two meanings for fear: apprehension in experiencing God's judgment and wrath when we fail to adhere to God's will, but also veneration, respect, and awe for God's wisdom, knowledge, and care for creation.

And *trust*? Why is it important to trust the Creator as essential for humanity? Trust is the belief in the truth, ability, reliability, and strength of the Creator that allows us to release ourselves into God's care. We, therefore, become the *stewards* rather than the *owners* of that creation. Most importantly, trust is addressed in the entire message of the Scriptures pointing to the restoration of a fallen creation through God's Son, Jesus.

A Working Definition of Humanness

So for the purposes of our discussion in this book moving forward, here is how I would define being a whole human being from a Christian, Scripturally sound perspective:

A fearing, loving, and trusting being created to be resilient by a loving and continuously engaged Creator with historically unified, integrated, yet individually unique body-mind-spirit natures, who possesses an awareness of God's law and will; the ability to love God, self, and others; and the capacity to trust in God's promise of restoration.

Please join me on this journey of wellness as a resilient human being as long as God grants us life on this earth.

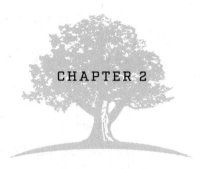

CHAPTER 2

LOSING RESILIENCE

I f we say being a human being is marked by resilience, then what does *resilience* mean in us and for us, especially as we grow older? A good definition of *resilience* is *springing back in shape.* Think of a *spring* or a strong, well-rooted oak tree like the one at the start of each chapter—it's a tree that generally returns to its shape and function despite powerful, disruptive storms. Another functional component of resilience, especially in nature, is the ability to recover *quickly* and *effectively* from threats and difficulties—to be *adaptable* to change.

Resilience

We can easily observe the characteristics of resilience in the physical world, as we look at things as common as machinery, clothing materials, or even in the elasticity of observable parts of our body like our skin. A material object that retains the ability to return to its baseline or adapt so that it can function optimally to face the next challenge is *resilient.* We'll explore in detail the physical resilience of our body and its organs in Chapter Four.

Increasingly, however, we are seeing the term *resilience* being utilized in the world of cognition and human behavior. A social scientist defines resilience as an individual's ability to successfully *adapt* to various life tasks in the face of social disadvantage or highly adverse conditions. Some of those *adaptive factors* include a positive attitude, optimism, the capacity to regulate emotions, and the ability to see struggles or failure as strengthening rather than a weakening force. A resilient person can have a positive outlook that allows them to adapt, change course, and continue forward. In contemporary parlance we might call resilient people *survivors.*

Behaviorally, possessing resilience becomes life-altering and life-prolonging as we face difficult circumstances such as the loss of a job or finances, loss of spouse or child, or the confrontation of serious illnesses like cancer, heart disease, Alzheimer's dementia, or trauma. Resilience is also helpful in the setting of relational problems or, especially these days, in the face of tragedies like loss of life or belongings due to natural disasters or terrorist attacks. Many people respond to such threats with a flood of debilitating emotions rather than healthy, resilient adaptation; this leads to a sense of uncertainty and instability. Cognitive or behavioral resilience is not just something that we are genetically born with, although we do see *resilient* families. Rather, behavioral resilience appears to be developed most commonly in an ongoing process that may require time, learning, and effort. Additionally, it may require a series of steps to accomplish.

Resilience does not imply that we humans are immune to distress physically, psychologically, or spiritually. We all experience emotional pain and suffering due to trauma in our lives. Although resilience generally is learned and developed, it may also, from a spiritual or faith perspective, be gifted to us through an undeserved and unearned relationship, particularly by a loving, ever involved God. We often admire individuals or families that seem to have a great ability to be resilient. Frequently, if you explore this resilience with them, they may tell you their resilience comes to a great extent from caring and supportive relationships within and outside of their social, familial, or faith *tribe*. Secure relationships are a primary factor in developing the ability to bounce back from adversity. More specifically, from my faith view, spiritual resilience is the result of the grace (free, favored) gift of my relationship with God provided through Jesus.

Looking closer, there are a variety of contributing factors that we associate with being psychologically resilient:

- A positive self-view; a confidence in your abilities and strengths
- The ability to develop realistic plans and to carry out steps to accomplish those goals
- The ability to solve problems and to communicate effectively
- The ability to manage strong or intense emotions, impulses, and feelings
- Faith; the intention and posture of turning yourself over or trusting in God's care and will to be best for you and your circumstances

Since emotional or behavioral resilience is often a developing process, there is a wide variation of strategies people use to achieve the ability to cognitively spring back from adversity. These patterns of response may grow out of cultural sensitivities and access to community resources. However, as I mentioned, an additional resource for resilience can be your family, social, or faith organization where you can actually gain personal resilience by being an integral part of a *helping community*.

Although you cannot avoid stressful events in your life, you may learn healthier ways to interpret and respond to these distasteful events. Or, due to losses and changes in your physical or social state, you may need to learn to adapt to your circumstances more effectively or quickly.

Resilient people can find smaller or more subtle paths to achieving bigger goals to accomplish on a more manageable, daily basis rather than feeling that they have to solve the entire problem in one fell swoop. Further, rather than lessening the stress they feel by detaching from a problem, they may learn to make decisive actions that move them forward, if ever so slightly.

There are a few more helpful strategies to build resilience:

- It is critical to keep every challenge in perspective, rather than blowing every distress into an unalterable, life-changing event.

- It is also imperative to learn something from each step in your response to stress and distress.

- It helps to be hopeful, constantly expecting good to be present simultaneously in whatever fearful distress you may be facing. When you are hopeful, you tend to take care of yourself. Seek activities and relationships that diminish stress and help you relax and calm yourself; eat well, exercise, and rest regularly. Reading, journaling, mediating, praying, and engaging in spiritual disciplines are all powerful resilience activities.

For many people, the sharing and actually giving over of physical, emotional, and, yes, spiritual distresses to God, can be the most important (and in the life of a person of faith) the quintessential response toward resiliency, especially as we age. In God's communication to us through the Scriptures, God invites us to place our distress into God's loving care rather than *solely* turning to our own abilities or strategies to face challenges. I think the best word to summarize this resilience-building behavior is still the word *trust. Trust God.*

Trusting, in no way, is merely a *coping mechanism* or a *detaching process.* We are human, the stresses we face are real, and distress can separate us from all we hold dear, including our own life. We are responsible and accountable to the choices we make and the circumstances of life in which we find ourselves.

However, the God who formed us also loved us so much that God gave us Jesus to restore the broken relationship brought about by our self-desires and self-driven choices. Christ died on the Cross to mend our torn relationship to a relational Creator, his Father. We receive this gift of healing and restoration of resilience purely by God's favor, by God's grace through our faith, not through our good deeds or our personal efforts. That faith is centered in our trust in Christ's substitutionary death in our stead. Christ's love-gift allows us to understand our renewed worth in God's eyes, permits us to make realistic goals and honorable purposes, opens the flow of communication to our God and those close to us, helps us understand and modulate our emotions, and constructs and strengthens our faith and trust in our Creator.

Homeostasis and Set-Points

If we have defined *resilience* as the ability to *spring back* to a state of readiness for the next threat to life and limb (and heart), then what *state* or *point* are we springing back to? What is the state of response in the body, thought, or relational being necessary to deal with what comes next? Scientists, psychologists, and philosophers have instructed us that in humans and much of nature, resilience allows us to return to *readiness* or *stability*, and we call that *homeostasis*. Homeostasis is critical after insult, and homeostasis returns us to a variety of *set-points* necessary to maintain life, particularly as a human creature.

Let's look at just a few biological systems in the human body and see how they work to regulate set-points and achieve homeostasis.

Body Temperature

Most of our core body temperature actually is controlled through the hypothalamus of the brain. When our temperature falls, the blood flow to our extremities and skin reduces. Blood is channeled into the trunk of the body where larger arteries exchange heated blood more directly to larger veins bringing that heat more quickly to our body's core. Our metabolism increases and then we may start to shiver to generate body warmth. On the other hand, when our temperature rises due to some trauma or infection, our skin sensors sense the heat and cause us to seek shade; we sweat, which when it evaporates, cools our skin and blood. We may increase our respirations (similar to panting in other animals), which cools the body through evaporation.[8]

Blood Sugar

All organisms regulate the concentration of glucose outside of their cells. Generally, in response to a rising glucose level, the *beta cells* of our pancreas secrete insulin and reduce the secretion of a substance called glucagon. This combined effect causes liver, fat cells, and muscle cells to use glucose more readily and convert the glucose into a stored format for later energy usage. Conversely, when the beta cells of the pancreas detect lower glucose in the blood, the beta cells decrease output and the neighboring pancreatic alpha cells are stimulated to pour glucagon into the blood. Glucagon stops the liver, fat cells, and muscles from taking up glucose from the blood. In fact, the liver is induced to start producing glucose that is dumped into the bloodstream correcting the shortage.

Blood Oxygen

The kidneys measure the oxygen content of arterial blood. When the blood oxygen levels are chronically low, kidney oxygen sensors secrete *erythropoietin* into the blood, causing the bone marrow to produce more red blood cells, which carry the oxygen supply in the bloodstream. This is why we might observe higher red blood cell concentrations in people living at higher altitudes (and why athletes from the University of Denver often seem to be able to outrun their rivals from the University of Iowa in long-distance races, especially when they run in the Rockies!)[9]

These are just a few of the multitude of homeostatic controlled systems within our remarkable bodies. Unfortunately, as the body ages, homeostasis and set-points can be substantially altered. With age, the efficiency of these control systems becomes diminished, which can bring about an unstable internal environment, illness, and physical changes in our bodies.

Similarly, as we age, the ability to maintain homeostasis in our cognition and our emotions decreases, although there is enormous individual variation. As complex as we might think biological systems are to achieve homeostasis, consider the complexity of the human mind in maintaining balance in the setting of self-esteem and the ability to set and achieve goals and respond to stress. The concept of homeostasis, therefore, also applies to perception, thought, comprehension, alertness, and particularly to behaviors, emotions, and relationships. However, rather than saying people are *psychologically homeostatic*, we might more commonly say that a person seems *well-balanced*, *stable*, or *even-keeled*.

Psychological homeostasis may be extremely hard to achieve or to sustain. Rather than thinking of *need states* in terms of bodily systems and function, in psychology we might think of *drive states*. Drive states are tougher to satisfy because they are affected by social expectations and cultural beliefs as well as internal psychological and biological capabilities.

For us as Christians, we also must consider spiritual and relational homeostasis, particularly as it applies to our loving relationship with God. From our faith perspective, we accept that there are internal as well as external forces at work to disrupt our relationship with our Creator, to destroy our ability to fear, love, and trust God. In a religious framework, we might apply the words *the devil, the world, and our own sinful flesh,* to characterize these forces which attempt to separate us from a fearing, loving, trusting relationship with our Creator

As a Christian, I believe that were it not for Jesus, I would not be able to have *homeostasis* with my Creator. In a real sense, Christ is our *set-point*. He restores the resilience, the homeostasis, the fear, love, and trust in God the Father, healing the damage of sin. Jesus permits me to approach God's throne of grace and mercy, allows me to be seen by God not as disordered but as ordered, not as diseased and blemished but as pure and worthy before the Creator. This is my faith and the basis of my resiliency.

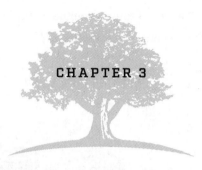

CHAPTER 3

MODELS OF RESILIENT AGING

The Blue Zones

It has been 500 years since there has been substantial, in-depth, and broadly researched writings on the *art* of living long, vibrant, and productive lives. However, we are living in fascinating times as interest in this topic is renewed in the 21st century. In 1550, the Italian Luigi Cornaro wrote a best-seller entitled *The Art of Living Long*. Cornaro proposed that you could extend the length of your life through practicing *moderation*; he lived into his nineties. Still, I would almost call that rather *contemporary* interest, in that we know many of the great, ancient philosophers and spiritualists who considered and advised their listeners on issues of aging well before the time of Christ.

In the last 17 years, however, a remarkable gathering of demographers, medical scientists, and journalists, under the banner of the National Geographic Society, are pursuing a strenuously arduous and meticulous study of five locations in the world where people are living not just longer, but with much less occurrence of many of the debilitating and life-limiting illnesses that we associate with aging—cancer, arthritis, and dementia, to name a few. They call these five areas of longevity *The Blue Zones*. I am most appreciative of the leadership and enthusiasm provided by Dan Buettner, primary author of this material, to whom I was first introduced at the Aspen Ideas Festival in 2016. I suspect you too might be familiar with Dan as he has appeared in numerous media formats.[10]

The Blue Zones

Ikaria
GREECE

Sardinia
ITALY

Loma
Linda
CALIFORNIA

Okinawa
JAPAN

Nicoya
Peninsula
COSTA RICA

What is so special about the name, *Blue Zones*? Nothing; it's just that as they were looking at these regions on a global map, the National Geographic team took a blue pen and circled five remarkable longevity spots on the globe, and *voila*, the Blue Zones.

These five regions—Ikaria, Greece; Sardinia, Italy; Okinawa, Japan; Nicoya Peninsula, Costa Rica; and Loma Linda, California in the USA—are identified by demographers to have an inordinate number of centenarians. Are people living to more than 100 by having access to extraordinary healthcare facilities, you know, lots of CAT scans, MRIs, Level One Trauma Centers, and board-certified specialty physicians? While that might be true of Loma Linda, with its magnificent Seventh Day Adventists medical facilities, most all of these communities just have good general public healthcare and good water supplies.

No, there must be something else at play to produce human beings with long, healthy, active lives. In fact, the scientists find nine common characteristics of life and living in the five blue zones. Here are nine common, healthy life skills or health habits characteristic of the nine zones:

- Natural Movement: The surrounding environment encourages people to move. People walk rather than ride. People use body movement to grow, harvest, and prepare their meals.

- Purpose and Mission: People have a purpose for getting up each morning, and it really isn't their "career" or "job." Having a purpose adds up to seven extra years to life. In fact, probably the greatest risk factor of dying in your mid-sixties in our western culture is *retirement.*

- Downshifting: People who live long know how to reduce the negative effects of stress by periodically slowing down, or downshifting, throughout the day. During these times their *stress-response system* (hypothalamus-pituitary-adrenal axis) slows down, stress secretions diminish, blood pressure lowers, and pulse rate decreases. They nap. They pray and meditate. They share a happy hour.

- 80% Rule: They stop their food intake when they sense their stomachs are 80% full. It is estimated that if we Americans follow this rule, we might lose as much as 17 pounds in the first year of our reduced intake.

- Plant-Slant: Innumerable studies show the tremendous benefit of following a predominantly vegetarian nutritional plan. Most centenarians eat little meat, but prefer beans as the cornerstone of their protein.

- Wine at Five: Centenarians, even a few of the Seventh Day Adventists, consume alcohol in moderation and with regularity. They imbibe one to two glasses of wine, generally not by themselves, but with food or friends.

- Right Tribe: In all of these cultures, a healthy cadre of friends helps to support healthy habits; they hold each other accountable. These friendship groups are committed to each other for life, through thick and thin.

- Spiritual Community: Regardless of religion or denomination, attending faith-based services approximately four times per month appears to add four to 14 years on to life expectancy.

- Loved Ones First: Prioritizing family above all else adds life and liveliness. Investing in children and grandchildren is empowering. Having a life partner or significant other adds significantly to longevity.[11]

Perhaps the most insightful finding from the Blue Zones is that you too can make long-term choices and behavioral changes in your personal environment that will gently nudge you to being more social, more mobile, less consuming, and more health conscious of what you are eating and drinking on a daily basis. Little changes can produce big benefits. And no matter when you start to make these life style changes, you may benefit. You just need to start *now*.

You may have very specific questions about the details of what seems to add vibrancy and longevity to life in the Blue Zones, and which health choices in food, friendship, or movement seem to pay the most dividends. I urge you to visit the appendix under *The Blue Zones Specifics* to explore further and to help develop pertinent strategies and wellness plans for yourselves and your families.

Since Loma Linda has the closest environment and demographics of any of the Zones for most of us, let me share a few thoughts on the Adventists' diet, which you may find helpful to your planning:

- Avocados are a terrific source of potassium, low in salt, and a great product to help reduce blood pressure and prevent strokes.

- Salmon, particularly wild caught, is filled with heart-healthy omega-3 fatty acids; try to consume 3-4-ounce servings a few times per week can reduce the chances of dying from a heart attack by a third. Since there is mercury, pregnant women might want to eat salmon once per week.

- Nuts (preferably non-salted) are a phenomenal snack and can reduce cholesterol, blood pressure, diabetes, chronic inflammation, and heart disease.

- Beans and lentils are great sources of protein daily and can replace much of the protein intake achieved by meat products.

- Clean, natural water, six to eight eight-ounce glasses per day, helps reduce consumption of sodas, fruit juices, and other high fructose added drinks in the diet. It is the easiest liquid for the body to process and flushes out the body's waste more efficiently than any other drink.

- Whole wheat bread is filled with nutrients and is far less caloric than other refined grains.

- Soymilk is used instead of other flavored varieties as an alternative to dairy. It has high protein, is low in fat, and contains phytoestrogens that are cancer protective. If available, goat milk and cheese products appear to be more digestible and less inflammatory to the gastrointestinal tract and immune system.

- Oatmeal, slow-cooked, is a breakfast staple in the Adventists' diet. It is loaded with fiber, iron, and B vitamins, and it fills you up.[11]

Can We Create a Blue Zone of Our Own?

Hearing this description of Blue Zones might lead you to ask, "Can we create Blue Zones within our own environment?" The National Geographic researchers believe this is indeed possible. Here are two of their fascinating and hope-building examples currently progressing in our country:[11]

- Southern California: There are three southern California towns— Manhattan Beach, Redondo Beach, and Hermosa Beach—where more than 23,000 people have made substantial lifestyle changes toward increased movement, meditation, and a plant-slant to their diets. Their commitments include walking three times per week; riding a bike for pleasure and transportation; learning new hobbies; setting aside a space and time for meditation, prayer, and quiet; and growing a garden. As a result, these Beach communities have seen a 17% reduction in smoking, a 50% reduction in childhood obesity, and $12 million dollars of savings in annual healthcare costs. Impressive!

- Spencer, Iowa: The town made a decision to redesign their community to make it more compatible to human movement and foot traffic; limit sprawl; assure easy access and reasonably priced vegetables; and provide plenty of access to gyms and playgrounds after school. In other Iowa towns, groceries added Blue Zone checkout lanes with healthy snacks; many restaurants added half-size portions and healthy sides to menus and created Walking School Bus routes and crossings. In a 2015 study by the Gallup organization, Iowa as a state moved from number 19 to number 14 in community wellness within five years. Impressive!

Based on Blue Zone research, here are other measures we can add to daily life to improve physical and mental resilience:

- Create a Blue Zone Kitchen: Place healthy ingredients in plain sight; equip your kitchen with utensils and cookware that encourage nonmechanized effort; lay out the kitchen in a triangle with the stove, sink, and refrigerator at the tips of the triangle, and have good light; use a smaller, energy-efficient refrigerator that is not overstuffed with food and keep a smaller pantry to discourage waste.

- Redesign your bedroom to encourage a good night's sleep: Buy a comfortable mattress and pillows; keep your thermostat between 62 and 65 degrees at night; keep your room dark during sleep and dim the room an hour before bedtime; keep your TV, computer, and cell phones out of the bedroom.

- Make your entire home a Blue Zone: Keep a scale in a prominent place and get on it regularly; keep one TV in your home and keep it normally out of sight to discourage mindless viewing, and hide the remote; move from power tools to hand tools; plant a garden and eat from it; walk a dog; ride a bike and walk; have one of your hobbies be sports; consider buying a few pillows or bean bag chairs to give your thighs an extra daily workout.

- Get into a social group, club, mutual care group, or actively participate in your faith community. Make note that people who belong to a faith-based community and attend community functions at least four times per month live four to 14 years longer than people who don't. Sing in the choir.

- Stop drinking soft drinks—and that includes diet colas and diet teas. Water, coffee, and natural teas clearly have been shown to have substantial health benefits including better blood flow, lower rates of Parkinson's and dementia, strong cancer prevention and anti-inflammatory properties, and, with red wine in moderation or with food, wonderful heart-healthy benefits.

- Snack on nuts; eat sourdough bread; eat beans daily; cut sugar; retreat from meat; reduce cow dairy by switching to soy/coconut/ almond or go sheep and goat's milk; have fish frequently, but in

3-4 oz. portions, and avoid predator fish like swordfish, shark, or tuna. Try to avoid farm-raised fish as they tend to be raised in crowded, antibiotic-treated, and pesticide-laden enclosures.

- Make absolutely certain that 95% of your diet is made up of plants; olive oil instead of butter; whole grains; soy for salt; low or no gluten; use leftover veggies to make soup or to freeze for a later use.[11]

We can do it, people! We can change our health behavior with individual, small, and nudging baby steps gradually incorporated into our daily habits. Each change in our movement, diet, rest, personal faith, and secular community's care for each other will have long-term benefits for all of us. We just have to *start*.

The *starting* is often the most difficult. How do we find motivation to move from apathy and inertia to animation and liveliness? Where do we find the courage and energy to change from physical, emotional, and spiritual funk to joy and abundant living?

I believe, physically, we can find motivation by taking a good, hard, and often difficult look at our current body function. Are we moving with ease and without distracting or limiting pain? Are we comfortable with our appearance, not just how we look in our clothes, but how we project our interest in others, especially our family? As we age, do we look and feel like a person who wants to be around for those who matter most in our lives— spouse, children, grandchildren?

Cognitively, intellectually, and emotionally, are we as bright and clear as we would like to be? Are we doing thinking activities that seem to help our memory, or are we forgetting dates and appointments and simple daily living tasks? Are our thoughts coming out in words easily and smoothly in our conversations with our loved ones?

Spiritually, are we finding our innermost thoughts to be ones of peace or of turmoil? What is our "self-talk" like? Is it harsh, accusatory, judgmental, or is it forgiving and calming?

If you are comfortable about where you *are,* it will be nearly impossible to change. And if you think you can accomplish change all by *yourself,* you are probably going to find your desired health behavior will be nearly impossible to *sustain.* You need community.

For some of us, that community will be family, those closest to us by marriage or genetics. I believe they are not just the motivating force for good self-care, but they are one of the main purposes for living and living functionally well. Those motivators also can be accompanied by friends and neighbors and even the communities we live in to sustain healthy patterns of movement, rest, and diet.

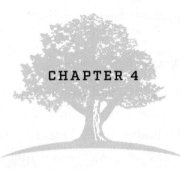

CHAPTER 4

CURRENT UNDERSTANDING OF PHYSICAL AGING— ALTERATIONS AND MAINTENANCE

We have examined what it means to be human. We have discussed the concept of human homeostasis, which seems to diminish or at least alter with aging. We have explored set-points of body, mind, and spirit. The general laws of nature appear to attack our ability to spring back responsively as we age. Let us now explore the specific types of change that occur in our *physical beings* and determine if there are options for us to help preserve function through proper stewardship of these gifts from our Creator.

In these next three chapters on physical, cognitive, and spiritual aging, I am going to dig fairly deeply and with substantial detail into specific age-related change. Perhaps, be prepared to dive in a bit more methodically. On the other hand, don't feel uncomfortable skimming over some of the "science stuff" and picking and choosing sections where you might have particular interest. You may always return to the details of a particular part of the body as questions arise.

I hope that the extra effort will pay dividends in understanding and preparation for sound health choices. In this chapter, I have tried to explain pertinent medical terminology, but if you still have specific questions, there is a substantial reference list at the end of the book.

Immunology of Aging

The headline for June 13, 2017, in the *Aspen Daily News*, another of our local papers, reads, "New Frontier in Cancer Care: Turning Blood into Living Drugs," by AP medical writer Lauran Neergaard.[12] The article describes a patient whose body was swollen with cancer, experienced treatment failures on top of treatment failures, and finally led to a highly radical approach and gamble. Doctors took some of the patient's immune cells and engineered them into cancer assassins and unleashed them into the patient's own bloodstream.

This approach of immune therapy is one of the most fascinating and hopeful frontiers in cancer care, actually creating "living drugs" that act as an army of tumor-seeking missiles to destroy cancer cells.

One of the most widely quoted earlier authors on the understanding of the aging immune system in humans is Takashi Makinodan in a text entitled *Biology of Aging: Retrospect and Prospect.* Dr. Makinodan defines aging as a "time-dependent process whereby one's body can no longer cope with environmental stress and change as easily as it once could." This loss of "physiological adaptability is one of the hallmarks of aging."[13]

As a primary care physician, I think it is appropriate to say that, as we age, we lose *immunologic resilience.* Let me now add some terminology and definition of the immune regulatory system to further our understanding and appreciation of this gift.

Our body contains *T cells.* T cells are key immune system soldiers standing guard to defend our body from foreign agents that could threaten health. But cancer cells, which are clearly foreign and health-threatening agents, can often still be difficult for our defense system's T cells to spot. Cancer cells can actually put the brakes on a defensive immune attack. Currently, one common immune therapy called "checkpoint inhibitors" can release one of the brakes on the T cells, allowing them to be more aggressive and effective defenders. The newer immune therapy approaches are actually giving patients stronger T cells to begin with.

Cancer currently kills about 600,000 Americans yearly, including 45,000 from leukemia and lymphoma, these being types of cancers particularly susceptible to immune therapy. We are in desperate need to expand the number of types of cancers that might be amenable to immunotherapy.

Substantial challenges to immune therapy remain, however. For example, living cancer drugs work for some people and some cancers but not for others. Furthermore, our physicians and scientists need to figure out how to manage potentially life-threatening side effects from an immune system that is "over-stimulated." Additionally, these types of therapies are basically made from scratch, customized, and at present, extraordinarily costly. This may represent *genetic engineering* at a most advanced stage.

We are quite early in this whole field of cancer research. While we remain extremely hopeful, there is much work to follow from some of the best of our medical researchers.

Genetic Markers of Aging

One of the more recent reviews of the immunology of aging comes from a 2014 text, *Immunology of Aging,* published by Springer, 2014, by Ahmad Massoud and Nima Rezaei (eds).[14] In an introduction by Mohamad Eslami, he begins by defining old age as the time of human life that lies between middle age and death; fair enough! In fact, the topic of how to quantitatively and qualitatively define old age could occupy an entire manuscript on its own merit. Suffice it to say that the transition to old age from earlier ages can be rapid in some individuals and more gradual in others. The pace of the transition seems to be related to both genetics and environment, as we have commented on earlier in the book.

As of this time there are no obvious and reproducible markers to identify the onset of old age. However, there is great interest among researchers in the length of *telomeres*, the nucleotide sequences (series of amino acids) that compose both tip ends of chromosomes. These tip ends appear to protect the chromosomes from shortening or eroding over time. We are aware that as we age and our cells reproduce repeatedly, the blueprints contained in the tip end of chromosomes (telomeres) tend to shorten.

Shortening of Telomeres in Aging

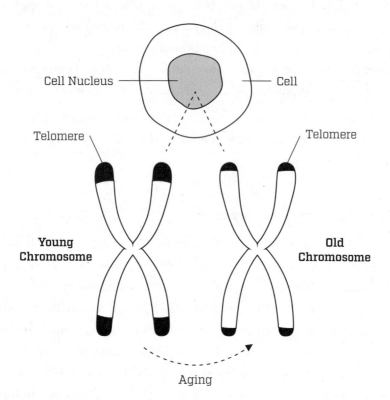

Cell Nucleus — Cell

Telomere — Telomere

Young Chromosome **Old Chromosome**

Aging

Our bodies possess an *innate* immune system made up of dendritic cells and macrophages, sort of the base camp for our protective system. But we also have a second component to protect us called an *adaptive* immune system, and major players in that system are T (as noted) and B lymphocytes. These cells replicate each time we face an insult with a resultant specific immune response. When these adaptive lymphocytes replicate, which is more often than the cells in the innate immune system, their telomeres shorten. Therefore the adaptive immune system will be far greater affected by aging and repeated threats to our health than the innate system.

The reality is that the as the immune system ages, it tends to become less effective as a protective barrier to the insults of environment and disease. Further, the immune system's effectiveness is dependent to a great extent on other organ systems in our bodies. The immune system loses its *resilience*.

One additional feature of our immunity: the various components of our immune system are often far apart and the components communicate with each other by a complex system of tiny secreted proteins called cytokines. Some cytokines that we often hear of are *interferon, interleukin, and tumor necrosis factors*. These proteins affect the behavior of other cells around them. Age alters these proteins and the receptors that pick up their signals in the cells. It is reasonable to say that as we age we develop a level of immunodeficiency.

However, is this *immunodeficiency* inevitable? I would suggest to a great extent it is *not immunologically* as dire as we might think. We know that there are many adults who actually age quite well, as I have referenced within the Blue Zones in Chapter Three, for example. These individual variations among heterogeneous (diverse) animals and humans may offer exciting new venues for exploration.

At current rates, this period of old age may extend over 30 years. Therefore it will be increasingly important to understand how our health choices either positively or negatively influence our immunity and how our immune system interacts and affects the other organs in our body that simultaneously may also be victims of aging.

We all know one obvious way an aging immune system displays itself clinically: aging adults are more susceptible to infections like influenza, shingles, pneumonia, bacterial and fungal skin infections, and the like. One area of preventive healthcare that certainly should be explored with your physician is the use of vaccinations for the more common and dangerous and potentially fatal illnesses. Influenza protection has been shown to have great value with the use of regular strength and so-called *senior strength flu* or *high-strength* vaccine for those over age 65.[15, 16]

Shingles, the painful blisters related to the dormant virus from previous chickenpox infection, may lie dormant for years and then reactivate. Shingles may affect one in three adults over age 50, and many physicians (including the US Communicable Disease Center or CDC) recommend a shingles vaccination for those over 50 where there is not a specific contraindication (primarily previous allergic reaction to components of the vaccine). Recently, a new, highly effective vaccine *SHINGRIX* (zoster vaccine recombinant, adjuvanted) has been released and appears to be the shingles vaccination of choice, even being recommended in those who have previously received herpes zoster vaccine.[17]

Finally, older adults over age 65 are far more susceptible to bacterial pneumonia particularly caused by pneumococcal disease, as are those 50 and older who suffer from diabetes or chronic heart and/or lung disease.[18]

Some of these vaccinations require two sequential doses, and all vaccinations should only be given after consultation with your primary care physician, as they understand best the risks and benefits of these therapies for you as an individual.

Nutrigerontology

Let me introduce you to a relatively vibrant newer area of medical study called *nutrigerontology*. Many people have had huge interest in this area for many years but it is now being recognized as having a significant place at the table of aging research.

Nutrigerontology is the study of the impact of nutrition, foods, macronutrient ratios, and diet on the aging process and lifespan. Much of this study is looking at the components of food and how those components affect inflammation in our bodies. It appears that much disease and certainly organ deterioration is related to the effects of inflammation. Can we select foods that assist our body in reacting and recovering from insults, whether chemical, infective agents like viruses, bacteria, or fungi, cancerous, or environmental? The answer is yes.

How fast are we aging? For the past 200 years, lifespans are increasing by three months/year in both sexes.[19]

What about the importance of dietary phytochemicals (non-nutrient compounds in plants) on inflammation and aging? There may be 4,000 or more phytochemicals in plants like fruits, vegetables, beans, and grains. Some commonly discussed phytochemicals include antioxidants, flavonoids, phytochemicals, catechins, polyphenols, and carotenoids.

Just a few better known phytonutrients include:

- Beta-carotene: Has a positive effect on immune system, vision, skin and bone. It is found in pumpkins, sweat potatoes, spinach, kale, and broccoli. Their colors are often orange and dark leafy greens.

- Lycopene: Affecting cancer (prostate) and heart health. It is found in tomatoes, pink grapefruit, watermelon, and red peppers. Heating these vegetables make the lycopene easier to absorb.

- Lutein: Good for eye health, cancer and heart health. Lutein is found in kale, spinach, broccoli, brussels sprouts, lettuce, and artichokes. Lutein is found in the macula of the eye.

- Resveratrol: Good for heart and lung health, inflammation, and cancer. Resveratrol is found in red wine, peanuts, and grapes. For example, one cup of red grapes can have 1.25 mgs of resveratrol.

- Anthocyanidins: Excellent for blood vessel health. It is found in blue and blackberries, plums, cranberries, red onions, strawberries, red radishes, and red potatoes.

- Isoflavones: Affects menopause, breast cancer, bone health, and joint inflammation, and helps lower cholesterol. The main vegetable containing isoflavones is soybeans. A half-cup of boiled soybeans contains 47 mgs of isoflavones.

Good general health, but in particular regular inclusion of phytonutrients, offers an active, preventive care strategy to add resilience to our immune systems in aging.[20, 21]

Pseudograins: Although this may not be the most appropriate location for a discussion of pseudograins (look and taste like grass grains and cereals—but aren't in that plant family), their value is real and I'll comment on them here.

- Amaranth—cultivated for more than 8,000 years by peoples like the Aztecs in Central America. These tiny golden seed have a nutty, creamy flavor and a comforting texture. Amaranth is an excellent source of iron and magnesium, calcium and fiber. It is the only grain known to contain Vitamin C.

- Buckwheat—in the rhubarb and sorrel family, this pyramid-shaped groat or kernel has a mild earthy flavor and was first grown in China and Japan. It is a great source of phytonutrients, and has lots of magnesium, soluble fiber, and can help control blood sugar.

Buckwheat has a high level of an antioxidant called rutin, which can help blood circulation.

- Quinoa—this pseudograin from spinach and Swiss chard has been called the "mother of all grains." It was gathered by the Inca. It also is nutty and earthy in flavor with a slight crunch. It is a great source of magnesium, fiber, folate, iron, and zinc. It also is colorful with red, black, and ivory varieties.

Pseudograins are complete proteins, meaning that their proteins have all of the essential amino acids in a healthy balance. This is because they contain at least 51 mgs of lysine per gram of protein; cereal grains do not. They are a wonderful protein source particularly for vegetarian diets. Check out the nutritional information in the *Environmental Nutrition* monthly subscription newsletter available at www.universityhealthnews.com under Health Publications.[22]

Gastrointestinal Tract in Aging

Gastrointestinal disorders and disease clearly increase with age. At least 40% of aged adults suffer at least one episode of age-related GI distress yearly. As a board-certified gastroenterologist, a number of GI disorders were common among my elderly patients.

Here's some of the so called "greatest GI hits" of aging!

Constipation

This is probably the most common GI disorder in the aged. There are numerous causes at the root of altered stool habits. Constipation may take the form of irregular or infrequent stools, painful bowel movements, and hard, dry stool. Constipation can be related to slower motility or movement of the muscular system in the GI tract that push digested food down the channel, and this allows more water to be reabsorbed, thereby drying the stool.

Commonly, older adults are on more medications that slow the GI system as a side-effect of the drugs. Calcium channel blockers that many people are on for heart or blood pressure disorders are extremely constipating. Of real concern are narcotic pain medicines critical to control the aches and pains of aging, particularly arthritis. These drugs dramatically affect motility.

Another cause of constipation is lack of water in the GI tract due to diuretics or even less oral fluid intake. Often we hesitate to drink more because we don't want to run to the bathroom to urinate as often.

The Effects of an Aging Liver

A comment should be made regarding the liver in aging and the effect on drug metabolism. Although there is known to be considerable variation of the effect of drug metabolism with age, generally aging impairs the biotransformation (alteration) of many drugs. Contributing to this are factors such as reduction in the total liver mass, hepatic enzymes diminishment in metabolizing capabilities, decreased blood flow in the liver, and alterations in plasma blood binding of drugs. However, it is often difficult to separate these effects from the fact that there are individual genetic variations in metabolic activity, concomitant disease effects, environmental factors, and dosage variations that all can have significant influence on the ways drugs are handled. An effective general strategy is to consider a slightly lower dose of drugs initially, and then adjust according to blood levels and effect. Much remains to be learned about this subject to improve drug therapy for many illnesses.[23]

GI Bleeding

The use of non-steroidal anti-inflammatory drugs (NSAIDs) that we use to control the inflammation of arthritis, make us at greater risk for gastrointestinal bleeding due to erosions and ulcers, particularly in the stomach. Dangerously, there may not be actual stomach pain from these types of erosions, but we may just experience black, tarry stools or even bright red blood in our bowel movements.

Diverticulosis

One fascinating disorder happening in nearly 50% of people over 60 is the development of small outpouchings or pockets in the lower gut or colon, called *diverticulosis*. These pockets are weakness in the wall of the colon and more often produce symptoms of gas, bloating, constipation, and diarrhea. However, these pockets can get inflamed and infected, producing fever and pain, and may require antibiotics, bowel rest, and occasionally surgery.

Swallowing Problems

Mouth and esophagus problems abound in aging. Poor dentition causes difficulty in swallowing, avoidance of some foods that might be highly nutritious, and chronic infection of teeth or gums with resultant painful chewing. The esophagus transports food from the mouth to the stomach; when it is disordered we may experience swallowing difficulties. This may be more prominent in people with dementia, strokes, Parkinson's disease, or other neurological disorders, all of which can affect swallowing.

Gastrointestinal Growths

Polyps (growths) anywhere in the GI tract increase with age particularly in the colon; they may have absolutely no symptoms or may cause bleeding or pain. Unfortunately, we know some of these polyps may be the precursors to colon cancer. In the past we identified age 50 with an increased risk of cancer occurrence, although we are seeing a dramatic increase in the incidence of colon polyps and cancer and especially rectal cancer in individuals in their 30s and 40s in this country. As of this writing, the American Cancer Society is now recommending beginning routine colon cancer screening at age 45 rather than 50. There are a number of ways this screening can be done: by stool blood or DNA testing, X-rays like CAT scans of the colon, or most commonly by colonoscopy. Colon screening definitely should be done before age 45 in people who have a family history of polyps or cancer. Continued colon cancer after age 75 should be discussed with your physicians to prudently weigh the risks and benefits of screening procedures. Studies show us that we can dramatically change colon cancer occurrence if we can remove polyps (growths) earlier in life.

Heartburn

In my experience, gastroesophageal reflux disease (GERD) or commonly called *heartburn*, may be the most common disorder of the aging GI tract. Just examine the volume of antacids (Tums and Gavison), H2 receptor antagonists (Tagamet, Cimetidine, Zantac), or proton-pump inhibitors or PPIs (Prilosec, Nexium, omeprazole) consumed in this country and around the world and you will get a quick sense of the frequency of this disorder, especially in old age. Often, obesity in aging contributes to GERD by increasing the pressure on the stomach pushing food, acid, and bile back up into the esophagus. Heartburn is the symptom marking much of this illness, but if untreated, the development of swallowing difficulties, pain, or even cancer can occur.

Dr. David Carr, noted internist and gerontologist at Washington University School of Medicine in St. Louis, shared with me in personal communication that some of the H2 receptor antagonists seem to have more significant anticholinergic effects (dry mouth, difficulty with urination) that the PPIs. However, the PPIs have also been associated with

B12 deficiency and mineral deficiency[24], which can be significant factors in the elderly, especially when these drugs are used on a chronic basis. There are also some reports of increased risk of pneumonia in the elderly on these drugs on a long-term basis.[25]

Incidentally, there are several reports surfacing to suggest that the chronic usage of medications like the H2 receptor antagonists or PPIs might be associated with increased risk of gastric cancer. Physician supervision and prudent usage of these medications, like all medications, is advised and you are urged to discuss further with your physician if you seem to require chronic use of these drugs to control heartburn or swallowing difficulties.

Gastrointestinal Tract Immune System

Finally, the gastrointestinal tract is a major part of our immune system, with lymph nodes and lymphatic channels filling the lining and walls of the gut. Our GI tract is definitely integral to both our *adaptive* and *innate* immune systems and the deterioration of these organ systems appear to contribute significantly to disease as we age.

Once again, we gradually lose our gastrointestinal resilience with age.

Proactive healthy choices for a resilient GI tract:

- Keep your teeth and gums healthy. Floss and brush; visit the dentist regularly; have your tongue and walls of the mouth monitored with each dental visit.

- Be aware of all the drugs you are taking, especially pain medications and NSAIDs. Consider taking aspirin or NSAIDs with food, or if you are susceptible to stomach ulceration, or under your physician's guidance, consider taking antacids or the acid-blocking agents. Furthermore, physicians may observe significant GI bleeding with older patients taking dual platelet therapy for stent placement or for prevention in stroke patients. Again, talk to your cardiologist or neurologist about this topic.

- Drink plenty of fluids. The 8 x 8 rule is still helpful: consume approximately 8 oz. of fluid, especially just plain old water, 8 times per day. Other liquids like milk, coffee, tea, or fruit juices can be counted as fluids, but good quality water is best.

- Exercise regularly; physical exercise definitely stimulates the GI tract. By exercise, we mean about 30 minutes of vigorous movement about five times per week. That's a good general rule and there is evidence this helps reduce colon cancer and risk of cardiovascular disease as well.

- Eat fiber, fiber, fiber! The increased fiber content in fruits and vegetables are an added benefit to all those phytochemicals. Fiber stimulates gut motility, helps hold on to fluid, and seems to benefit diverticulosis and possibly even improve cancer risk. The average male should take in at least 35 grams of fiber and the female at least 25 grams. Eat *whole* foods like multigrain or whole wheat. Since *high fiber* cereals can sometimes be tasteless, mix with your favorite cereal. Consider oatmeal, especially steel cut oats, for great fiber. Move to brown rice rather than white rice; it is chewier and nuttier. Try eating the actual fruit rather than always juicing; you usually will consume less sugar and increase your fiber intake in this way. If you love OJ, get the ones with added pulp. Try granola, either as the full cereal serving or just sprinkled on top. Start consuming beans (remember the Blue Zones where everyone seems to stay healthier with a cup of beans a day). Use veggies for snacks, especially peppers, carrots, celery, and broccoli; add a low-calorie dip. Consider nuts for snacks or even try air-popped popcorn and try not to goop it up with salt and butter.

- Manage your weight. Obesity is a major contributor to GERD, but we also see studies demonstrating an increased risk of colon cancer with obesity. Simultaneously, remember that you are decreasing risk and difficulty in controlling diabetes, heart disease, and high blood pressure.

- Probiotics are a major area of both medical science and media/ marketing interest these days. The normal and healthy GI tract is filled with bacteria and yeast, some helpful and others deleterious; balance of the various types is critical. Naturally good bacteria can be obtained in foods such as yogurt, chocolate, and fermented vegetables like sauerkraut and miso. But these foods are not always a part of many American diets...well, except for chocolate. Our routine diet might be altered when we travel, consume medications or antibiotics, or experience stress; an unhealthy diet can drastically change the balance of organisms in our gut.

There is increasing interest in probiotic supplements that have a variety of Bifidobacterium (found in the large bowel or colon), Saccharomyces boulardii (Brewer's Yeast), a good yeast, and lactobacillus (small intestine inhabitants).

Probiotics seem to help move food through the gut. They appear to have particular benefit for people with irritable bowel syndrome (IBS), inflammatory bowel disease (IBD), infectious diarrhea due to bacteria, viruses, or parasites, or antibiotic-related diarrhea. They may also help with eczema, genitourinary health, allergies, and oral health, according to some reports. It is imperative that you consult your doctor about appropriate probiotics for your specific condition as probiotic supplements are not generally regulated by the FDA nor are they formally endorsed by any physician professional organizations at this time.

Finally, get regular GI tract screenings, including colonoscopies on a regular basis at and after age 45, and at earlier ages if you carry a family history of colon cancer or polyps. Definitely see your family doctor and gastroenterologist if any GI symptoms develop.

A resilient GI tract makes one healthy, wealthy, and wise—or something like that!

Endocrine System in Aging

The endocrine system is made of organs and tissues throughout the body that produce *hormones*. Hormones are naturally produced chemicals that are made at one site in the body, released into the bloodstream, and then are able to influence other target organs and cells in the body at distant locations.[26]

Hormones influence their target organs; but it is important to note that some organs have their own internal control system, along with or instead of hormones. Aging affects these hormonal and internal control systems. Some organs desensitize to hormones. Sometimes the total quantity of the hormones decreases.

In aging, the blood levels of some hormones increase, and some decrease. Further, the way the hormones are metabolized or broken down may slow in aging.

To state this differently, the pattern of both endocrine hormone secretion and target organ receptivity are altered in unique ways in aging. Here are a few examples.

Vasopressor hormones, often affecting the cardiovascular system, both *increase* (norepinephrine) and *decrease* (renin and aldosterone) in aging. Renin causes an increase in blood pressure to restore perfusion pressure in the kidney, and aldosterone affects blood pressure and causes the bloodstream to reabsorb water with sodium to increase blood volume. The kidney hormone renin stimulates the adrenal gland to release aldosterone.[27]

Let's look at a few specific examples of hormone-secreting endocrine tissues. You might recall from science or psychology class (or if you read my book *Fear, Anxiety and Wellness*) that stress stimulates the HPA-axis (hypothalamus-pituitary-adrenal-axis), which leads to the well-known *fight or flight stress response*. In the base of the brain, at the forefront of this stress-response, is the *hypothalamus*. The hypothalamus secretes hormones that stimulate the pituitary gland (also at base of the brain) and the adrenal glands (lying just above the kidneys).

HPA-Axis

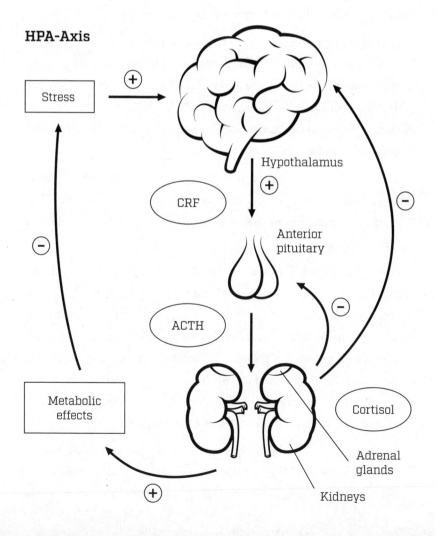

In aging, the absolute amount of hormone being produced by the hypothalamus remains about the same, but the responsiveness of the target organs diminishes.

The next in line, the pituitary gland, actually changes in size as we get older. It is the largest in middle age, but then begins to diminish in size. The pituitary has two parts: the *posterior* part stores the hormones secreted by the hypothalamus; the *anterior* part produces the hormones that target and control the thyroid gland, growth, the cortex of the adrenal gland, and the testicles, ovaries, and breasts—pretty important stuff!

The thyroid gland controls our metabolism, the rate at which we utilize energy. With aging the thyroid gland can develop lumps or nodules; starting at age 20, our metabolism begins to slow. Generally, thyroid hormone levels in the blood remain stable, but sometimes the levels begin to rise; this leads to increased cardiovascular risk and is why cardiologists will often check thyroid hormones as part of your checkup.[28]

Four small glands adjacent to the thyroid are the parathyroid glands. They control the level of calcium and phosphorus essential for bone strength. Parathyroid hormone levels tend to rise with age, contributing significantly to *osteoporosis*.

The pancreas produces *insulin* that helps glucose enter into cells for energy. Cells become less sensitive to insulin with aging, especially after age 50. However, not only do we seem to have less insulin from the pancreas as we age, we tend to develop so-called *insulin resistance*. This means that the ability of blood insulin to dispose of glucose in our blood can diminish, so our blood concentration of glucose increases, with many adverse effects on our metabolic function. We know this also happens in people who are obese and certainly with those with adult onset diabetes.

In aging, our body tends to increase in weight and fat mass, especially around our belly and hips, and these factors definitely contribute to the development of insulin resistance. The good news is that diet, weight reduction, and exercise all help delay insulin resistance and may also help delay or prevent the development of diabetes.

In terms of dramatic bodily function, the distal end of the HPA-axis, the *adrenal* glands, sit just on top of the kidneys. The adrenal glands also have two sections with different functions. The outer layer, called the *cortex*, produces aldosterone, cortisol, and dehydroepiandrosterone. Aldosterone regulates fluid and electrolyte levels in the bloodstream. Aldosterone decreases with age and the decrease can lead to *orthostatic hypotension,* or sudden passing out we see in elderly when they suddenly stand up from a sitting or lying position. Cortisol is the "stress hormone" and it affects the metabolism or breakdown of fat, protein, and glucose. It also has anti-inflammatory and anti-allergy effects. Even though cortisol secretion decreases with age, the blood levels remain roughly constant. Dehydroepiandrosterone levels also decrease with age, but the result of this drop is not clear.

Another part of the endocrine system is also part of our reproductive organs: testes and ovaries. The testes and ovaries have two functions. They produce sperm and eggs, respectively. But they also produce the sex hormones that control facial hair and breasts. Aging men can have lower testosterone levels and aging women experience less estradiol and estrogen post menopause.[29]

In summary, the following hormones tend to decrease with age:

- Renin
- Aldosterone
- Calcitonin
- Growth hormone
- Estrogen and prolactin often decrease in women

Hormones that tend to remain roughly the same in aging include:

- Cortisol

- Epinephrine

- Insulin

- T3 and T4 thyroid hormones

Hormones that tend to increase levels with age are:

- Parathyroid hormone

- Norepinephrine

- LH or luteinizing hormone

- FSH or follicular-stimulating hormone

Our appropriate balancing of hormones affects innumerable organ systems and function to add resilience to our whole, healthy beings.

Tissue in Aging

All living tissue is made up of cells, and all of our body's cells share some similar characteristics, although they do not all have the same function. Layers of cells that have similar function are called *tissue*. Different types of tissues grouped together make up organs. An organ is a part of an organism that is typically self-contained and has a vital function (e.g., brain, kidney, liver, or heart).

There are four basic types of tissues:

Connective tissue: This is supporting material that holds together various organs. In this group are blood, bone, lymph tissue, and the tissues that give structure and provide support internal organs and skin.

Epithelial tissue: This covers deeper body layers. The skin and the internal linings of organs like the gastrointestinal tract are made of epithelial tissue.

Muscle tissue, including three types:

- Striated muscles or voluntary muscles that move the skeleton

- Smooth muscles or involuntary muscles that line the stomach and other internal organs
- Cardia muscle (also involuntary) that makes up most of the heart

Nerve tissue: This makes up the neurons or nerves that carry communications to various parts of the body. The brain, spinal cord, and peripheral nerves are made of nerve tissue.

Returning to the body's cells, we understand cells to be the basic building blocks of the body. As they age they become larger and less capable of dividing and multiplying—they become less *resilient*.

Fatty substances and pigment increase within the cells and they function less efficiently or abnormally. Waste builds up within the cells resulting in the buildup of dark material called lipofuscin. Eventually cells die; they cease to carry out their function within the body.

Cells die either because they naturally get old and are replaced by new cells, or they may succumb to disease, injury, or the death of the organism of which they are a component. We divide cell death into two basic types: programmed cell death (PCD) and autophagy.

Programmed cell death, or Type I cell death, is highly regulated and actually confers an advantage to the body's life-cycle. One example of this regulated death is the cells that embryonically form between our toes or fingers; these cells *apoptose* (cease to live; kind of committing suicide by the cells) and we then have separated digits. On the other hand, Type II cell death (autophagy or self-devouring) is another form of regulated cell-death, which allows the destruction of some parts of the cell and the use of other parts of the cell to rebuild the cell.

Cell death, as mentioned above, can also be due to extra-cellular factors like infection or trauma; we call these processes cellular *necrosis* or *necroptosis*. Finally, since we deal with so much cancer in this world, we understand that cancer cells can be made to prematurely or inappropriately enter the process of *mitosis* (replicated chromosomes separating into two new nuclei) due to our treatments for that cancer (such as giving ionizing radiation therapy), and subsequently destroy the cancer cell. We call this cell-death *mitotic catastrophe*.[30] While we are talking about cancer cells, there is one further cell death caused by several cancer drugs and we call that *paraptosis*. That's desired; that's good.

So some cells in their life-style die completely, and some just suffer intracellular changes that make them less effective or functional. Connective tissue loses resilience and becomes stiffer, less elastic. Therefore the organs, blood vessels, and lung tissue containing connective tissue become rigid. The membranes of the cells actually weaken, making it harder to supply oxygen and nutrients to the cell for energy and making it more difficult for the cell to dispose of waste and carbon dioxide. The cell becomes starved and poisoned. Some tissue atrophies or loses mass and some become lumpy and stiffer.

Since we rarely use our organs fully, and since these aging changes occur slowly, we often don't immediately notice these highly significant changes in structure and function.

Probably the most detrimental tissue changes happen in our heart, lungs, and kidneys, and we will examine those in more depth in a moment. Major changes also occur in the cells of our brains and nervous system and we will devote Chapter Five to those topics. However, all the organs and systems in our body are interrelated and highly interdependent to work as a whole. Occasionally our body and mind are asked to work harder than usual under certain trying circumstances. Some of these times might be when we are ill, when we are required to take certain medications, when we are under substantial or prolonged stress of body, mind, or spirit. But we also work harder when we are exposed to the demands of increased exertion or higher altitude. Parts of our body or the whole body itself may fail, leading to substantial dysfunction or death.

As our body has less resilience or reserve capability, our response to drugs can alter significantly. We might require higher or lower doses of medications to function properly. Side effects of the medications can mimic actual diseases and so we mistake a drug reaction for a real disease. We are all aware of situations where an older person reacts far differently than a younger person with a given dose of medicine.

Cellular Changes in Aging

We have a variety of ways of describing what happens to cells with aging:

Atrophy: Cells shrink in size and as a result, organs may decrease in size. We see this in bone, muscle, the heart, and sexual organs. It is not clear what causes this but contributing factors include less use, less workload, less blood supply and nutrients to the organs, and reduced stimulation from hormones and nerves.

Hypertrophy: Occasionally cells or organs increase in size with age. This is caused by increases in the amount of protein in the cell structures or its lining membrane rather than fluid increase in the cell. Sometimes when cells in one part of the organ or body atrophy, others hypertrophy to make up for the loss of total cell mass.

Hyperplasia: To compensate for decreased cell size, function, or number, cells may increase the rate of replication. We see this in skin after an injury, or in the bone marrow, or gastrointestinal tract. The liver, for example, can regenerate 70% of its volume within two weeks after injury. That's why we can transplant a small portion of liver into a person with liver failure and have it regenerate almost full liver function in short order.

Dysplasia: The shape, size, or organization of some cells can proceed abnormally. This can happen in the cervix or the respiratory tract.

Neoplasia: Cells can form tumors that can be benign (noncancerous) or malignant (cancerous). Malignant cells can reproduce quickly and with abnormal shape or function.[31, 32, 33]

So is it *nature* (genetic blueprints in our cells) or is it *nurture* (our diet, ultraviolet light, wear and tear on tissue and organs, accumulation of metabolic waste) that determines the effects of aging in connective tissue? Most scientists, physicians, and gerontologists (people who specialize in the study and treatment of aging) agree that it is all of the above, with nature and nurture doing an interactive dance yielding varying results on lifespan and quality of life. That quality of life (being nimble or being frail in aging) will be taken up in more depth as we get into a discussion of our muscles, joints, and bones in a moment.

The Face in Aging

Perhaps because we communicate by looking directly at each other (well, hopefully this is the case despite electronic communication devices, texting, and voicemail), changes in the appearance of our faces are most notable in the aging process.

The skin of our face and neck may droop or sag or even fall over itself, resulting in the dreaded double chin. In aging, our skin becomes thinner, and muscle tone lax. The skin becomes drier, and the fat layers that support the skin may lessen, so the surface wrinkles. Damage due to sun or cigarette smoking speed these changes. Dark facial blotches are usually due to sun damage; however, some women experience dark blotching of the skin beginning in pregnancy; these discolorations can become prominent feature of their faces as they age.[34]

Loss of teeth and gum tissue can bring about a gaunt or sunken appearance. If we lose bone mass in the jaw, it may make our nose, forehead, or eyes appear abnormally prominent. Your nose may actually lengthen— and it is not just due to lying about your age, Pinocchio!

Your ears may lengthen due to cartilaginous growth, and men particularly may develop coarse, dark, long hair within the ear. Wax tends to lessen as sebaceous glands diminish, and if the remaining wax hardens it can diminish hearing.[35]

Eyelashes and eyebrows turn gray. Wrinkles or crow's feet develop around the eye socket. Eyelid fat may sink below the eye creating bags and making the eyes look more sunken. Vision can be affected by drooping of the upper eyelids.

The cornea or outer surface of the eye can turn gray; the iris or colored portion of the eye can lighten making the aged appear to have pale or blue-gray eyes.[36]

No wonder we look different with age!

Skin in Aging

I have mentioned changes in the skin of the face as we considered the facial alteration occurring with age. Let us look at the whole skin surface as our skin is most critical in preserving resilience in aging of many internal organs.

The skin has many purposes:

- It helps preserve the fluid and electrolyte balance of the body.
- It forms a protective coat to shield internal structures from injury due to infectious agents, sun, and chemical exposure.
- It is filled with nerve receptors that allow you to sense the environment.
- It helps control your body temperature.

The skin is made up of three layers:

- Epidermis: this outermost layer contains skin cells, pigment, and proteins.
- Dermis: this is the middle layer holding blood vessels, oil glands, nerve cells, and hair follicles and its purpose is to provide nutrients to the epidermis.

- Subcutaneous layer: this innermost layer contains fat, additional blood vessels and hair follicles, and sweat glands.

Holding all three layers together is connective tissue filled with collagen and this provides the flexibility, elasticity, and support for the strength of the skin.

So what happens to our skin and how does the appearance of it change as we age? As I have mentioned, probably the greatest threat to our skin is sun exposure. However, environmental factors like makeup, chemicals and soaps, nutrition, smoking, and our genetics all have an influence on this protective barrier.

Darker-skinned people tend to tolerate sun damage better than light-skinned, blue-eyed folks, due to increased pigments that provide some protection.

The first change that comes with age is a thinning of the epidermis, although the number of skin cells remains roughly the same.

Melanocytes, the pigment containing cells, decrease in number but actually expand in individual size. This makes the skin appear more translucent and creates the appearance of so-called age spots or liver spots.

The skin's strength and elasticity decrease and is especially noticeable in sun-exposed regions producing the leathery farmer's tan seen in people who work outside much of their lives.

Blood vessels in the dermis layer become fragile and easily bleed and bruise or may appear to *bubble* in the well-recognized, tiny, cherry hemangiomas.

Even the fatty or sebaceous level is affected as the oil glands produce less oil, thereby producing dry, scaly skin. Also, with the loss of the sebaceous fat, there is a loss of insulation, and so many elderly tend to complain of hypothermia in cold weather. Sweat glands in this layer also diminish so it is harder to dissipate heat.

Finally, there tend to be more unsightly skin tags and warts.

With a thinner, more fragile, less elastic and less sensitive skin, injury increases and repair or resilience diminishes. Relatively minor trauma can lead to major bruises, tears, and blood collections called *purpura* (large purple-red blotches). Sadly, illnesses like diabetes, immune disorders, and lessened blood flow due to hardened arteries, liver disease, obesity, and adverse reactions to medications all contribute to this decreased resilience and less efficient self-repair.

Public awareness is dramatically heightening as we recognize the increase in skin cancer in aging from previous sun exposure. This includes all skin cancer: basal cell, squamous cell, and melanoma.[37]

What can we do to add resilience to aging skin?

- Use high PABA (4-aminobenzoic acid) skin protection to avoid sunburn and begin this in your babies and children. However, continue this at any age. Wear hats and clothing especially that may contain sun-block products.[38]

- Avoid smoking, which causes the release of an enzyme that breaks down collagen and elastin, both important components to skin health.

- Get sleep, because when you don't get adequate sleep your body produces excessive cortisol that can break down skin cells. Conversely, when you sleep enough, you produce more human growth hormone (HGH), which helps the skin remain thick and elastic.

- Eat more fish, particularly salmon with its good protein and excellent omega-3 fatty acids. This keeps the skin plump and youthful. Also, eat more soy, which seems to heal some of the damage due to the sun.

- Drink cocoa on occasion instead of coffee (this will make my wife very happy). Cocoa contains two excellent dietary falvanols (epicatchin and catechin) that can protect the skin from sun damage and improve skin hydration.

- Eat lots of fruits and vegetables with their wonderful antioxidant compounds.

- Finally, moisturize with good-quality lotions and avoid heavily perfumed soaps that dry the skin. Be extremely careful with bath oils, which can be extremely slippery and cause falling. Simultaneously, try not to over wash the skin and dry it out. Look for products with AHAs, which are natural fruit acids that can lift away the top layer of dead skin cells, especially around the eyes, and reduce wrinkles. AHAs may also stimulate collagen production.

Furthermore, you may also consider trying Retin A, which is only obtained by prescription, which does have side-effects of burning of the skin and hypersensitivity, or you might be able to get retinol, a natural form of Vitamin A found in over-the-counter products.

There is also some evidence that Vitamin C can increase collagen production and provide some protection from UVA and UVB rays; it may also correct pigmentation problems and improve eczema or other skin irritations.

There are also a host of "medical/spa" treatments for aging skin that are heavily advertised in the media. These include the use of Botox (Botulinum toxin A injections), which relaxes muscle just under the skin and reduces the wrinkles. There are also wrinkle fillers including collagen and hyaluronic acid. There are laser/light resurfacing treatments from a laser or pulse diode light, all of which wound the skin and kick collagen into high gear. Furthermore, there are a variety of chemical peels to burn away the top layer of skin, and dermabrasion to bring a more even texture to skin surface. All of these should be used in the hands of skilled and professionally accredited physicians, as they all may have significant side effects.[39]

Male Reproductive System in Aging

The male reproductive system tends to change gradually rather than more suddenly as occurs in women. Rather than *menopause* (women), men's changes can be referred to as *andropause*. The main changes occur in the testes, where testicular mass tissue diminishes and testosterone levels gradually lessen. It may be increasingly difficult for men to maintain an erection, but this too happens gradually; it may begin as a lack of nocturnal involuntary erections but becomes greatly concerning when seeking purposeful erection. In addition to the natural course of aging, multiple medical disorders and medications, as well as psychological issues, may contribute to erectile dysfunction (ED) in aging.[40]

There are two primary areas where the male reproduction system demonstrates loss of resilience in aging:

- Fertility: The tubes that carry sperm can develop sclerosis (narrowing), or a loss of elasticity. Although sperm continue to be produced, the rate of production diminishes. Key components of this system such as the epididymis, seminal vesicles, and prostate continue to produce fluid critical to carrying sperm forward, but their surface cells diminish.

- Urinary function: In aging men, the prostate gland tends to enlarge, sometimes to substantial size, obstructing the flow of urine. Some of the normal prostate tissue is replaced by scar tissue and this process is called *benign prostatic hypertrophy* (BPH). This probably affects up to 50% of aging men. Additionally, this benign enlargement may interfere with ejaculation.

What are the effects of these changes on reproduction and urinary function? Age does not predict fertility per se, and fertility varies among men of a given age. Nor does prostate function specifically affect fertility. After removal of the prostate gland (*prostatectomy*), men can still conceive children and fairly older men can also be fathers. Even though the amount of fluid in the ejaculate might seem about the same, the number of living and functional sperm diminishes with age.

Older men may have a lower libido or sex drive. They may also be slower to respond to stimulation. Although this can be due to lower testosterone levels, issues such as co-existent illnesses, lack of willing partners, medications, chronic conditions like heart or lung disease, or psychological stresses like anxiety or depression, may be substantial factors in ED.

ED is a highly recognized disorder in males and the focus of tremendous discussion in the media, pharmaceutical, and scientific community. Sales of medications to treat this disorder are brisk. Most commonly, ED is due to concurrent medical conditions or medications themselves, rather than just aging alone; perhaps 90% of ED is medically rather than psychologically based. Two of the most common conditions are due to medications to treat hypertension, and the development of diabetes. Fortunately, these causes may well be treatable and reversible.

Benign prostatic hypertrophy causes the drainage tube from the bladder to the urethra to be partially obstructed. Men may struggle to urinate or empty their bladder adequately. Men with BPH may be able to tell you every restroom in their neighborhood. BPH may lead to repeated urinary tract infections, kidney failure, and prostatic infection or *prostatitis*.

Of course, we cannot leave the discussion of the aging male reproductive tract without a mention of prostate cancer with, perhaps, one of every five to six men experiencing this malignancy in their lifetime. In addition, benign and malignant tumors of the bladder may occur, often with bleeding, and occasionally with very difficult and tragic results. In younger men, testicular cancer may be of greater risk than prostate cancer.[41]

However, prostate cancer does occur in younger men, so awareness of this malignancy is valuable in all males, especially if there is a family history of prostate cancer. Appropriate prostate cancer screening includes regular digital-rectal exams and PSA (prostatic specific antigen) blood tests, beginning at age 50 in all men, and earlier with a family history or specific urinary symptoms. If you have more interest in this subject, consult your primary care physician or urologist and also follow up-to-date guidelines at the National Cancer Institute's website, www.cancer.gov and explore *psa-fact-sheet*.

There is much media emphasis on various supplements and remedies for the treatment of erectile dysfunction and enhancing male fertility. Nonetheless, prostate cancer, prostatic enlargement, and testicular atrophy (all which can lead to erectile dysfunction and reduced fertility) are *not* preventable diseases. Early and proactive diagnosis and management of these disorders is imperative.

Finally, there are many proponents in the medical community and non-medical community who suggest that measuring testosterone levels and providing supplements that will help build bone and muscle, help memory, prevent falls, etc. in older men. I believe the final word is still not in. I think we can say that supplementing testosterone does not seem to improve cognition and may even increase cardiovascular disease.[42] As I have said before, thorough consultation with your primary care physician and/or urologist will allow you to balance the risks and benefits of these therapies.

Kidneys and Bladder in Aging

The kidneys have a vital detoxification and fluid balance function in the body. They filter waste from the blood and remove excessive fluid. They also help control the chemical and acid-base balance in the body.

The kidneys lie at the top of a system that includes the ureters that connect the kidneys to the bladder and the urethra which empties the bladder. Muscular changes in the body can affect bladder control and emptying.[43]

With aging, the kidneys lose total mass, the filtering units called nephrons diminish, and blood vessels may harden, which causes slowed filtration of the blood.

The walls of the bladder too may change, becoming less elastic or resilient, unable to stretch, and therefore able to hold less urine. Furthermore, the muscles of the bladder can weaken, making the bladder harder to empty. Finally, the urethra can become obstructed in men, as we have mentioned, due to an enlarged prostate. In women, prolapse or falling of the bladder or vagina can impede urine flow. As always, medications and co-existent illnesses may affect renal function.[44]

Chronic kidney disease, repeated urinary tract infections, and bladder leakage (incontinence) or urinary retention (inability to completely empty the bladder) are common in aging.

There are several symptoms that should prompt you to seek medical attention especially as you age:

- Dark or bloody urine
- Difficulty in urinating or frequent urination
- Burning upon urinating
- Urgency in urination
- Signs of infection including fever and chills, burning, nausea, and vomiting, lower back pain, or severe fatigue[45]

Of particular note in the list above is the difficulty or hesitancy in urination caused by drugs rather than tissue obstruction; this may be a common issue for men (but also women) taking common anticholinergic medications like cold remedies (antihistamines, Zyrtec, or Chlor-Trimeton); antispasmodics for stomach disorders (Levbid or Ditropan);

and some tricyclic antidepressants to treat anxiety and depression (Elavil, for example).

A final suggestion for men is to be aware of a number of male reproductive and genitourinary health screening questionnaires to assist men in screening for disorders. The American Urological Association Symptom Score (AUASS) is a simple questionnaire to help you assess the severity of an enlarged prostate gland. It is readily available on line at www. urologix.com. One note of caution is that symptoms of enlarged prostate can easily be confused with prostatic cancer, and therefore, consultation with your primary care physician and urologist for a full discovery of the cause of you symptoms is imperative and should not be delayed.[46]

Female Reproductive System in Aging

Aging in the female reproductive system is primarily a result of hormonal changes and the onset is signified by *menopause,* in which the menstruation or periods cease to occur on a permanent basis.

Menopause is often signaled by a time of more frequent, missed, or irregular periods, heavier or lighter flow, and longer or shorter length of menstrual periods. This is called *perimenopause*, and it may begin several years before the last period. Along with these menstrual changes come changes in the woman's menstrual tract and physical appearance, also hormonally related.[47]

- Menopause usually occurs between 45 and 55.

- The ovaries cease to make estrogen and progesterone.

- The ovaries stop making eggs and it is no longer possible to get pregnant.

- Menstrual bleeding stops—but to be safe, a woman should continue birth control for at least a year after the last period if she wishes to avoid pregnancy.

- If bleeding occurs after one year without periods, this is abnormal and should be immediately evaluated by the gynecologist.

- Vaginal walls become thinner and drier and sexual activity may become uncomfortable or painful.

- You may become more susceptible to vaginal yeast infections.

- The external genitalia can become thinner and more irritated.

- Symptoms of moodiness, hot flashes, headaches, and insomnia may increase.

- Breast size may decrease.

- Short-term memory may diminish.

- The muscles of the pelvis may weaken leading to a tilting or dropping of the uterus, bladder, or vagina called *prolapse.*[48]

Help for Female Changes with Aging

Since hormonal changes are at the core of the changes, hormonal therapy also is the hallmark of help. The addition of appropriate doses of estrogen or progesterone may help in reducing hot flashes, painful intercourse, and vaginal dryness. Painful intercourse also may be helped by lubricants and moisturizers that can be purchased over the counter. Vaginally applied estrogens may help thicken the vaginal wall and improve moisture levels.[49]

The topic of hormone replacement therapy for women has many considerations, proponents and opponents. A recent recommendation from the North American Menopause Society follows:

> *Hormone therapy (HT) remains the most effective treatment for vasomotor symptoms (VMS) and the genitourinary syndrome of menopause (GSM) and has been shown to prevent bone loss and fracture. The risks of HT differ depending on type, dose, duration of use, route of administration, timing of initiation, and whether*

a progestogen is used. Treatment should be individualized to identify the most appropriate HT type, dose, formulation, route of administration, and duration of use, using the best available evidence to maximize benefits and minimize risks, with periodic reevaluation of the benefits and risks of continuing or discontinuing HT.

For women aged younger than 60 years or who are within 10 years of menopause onset and have no contraindications, the benefit-risk ratio is most favorable for treatment of bothersome VMS and for those at elevated risk for bone loss or fracture. For women who initiate HT more than 10 or 20 years from menopause onset or are aged 60 years or older, the benefit-risk ratio appears less favorable because of the greater absolute risks of coronary heart disease, stroke, venous thromboembolism, and dementia.

Longer durations of therapy should be for documented indications such as persistent VMS or bone loss, with shared decision making and periodic reevaluation. For bothersome GSM symptoms not relieved with over-the-counter therapies and without indications for use of systemic HT, low-dose vaginal estrogen therapy or other therapies are recommended.[50]

In other words, always consult your primary care physician or OB-GYN who knows you well and understands all of your health challenges before embarking on the use of hormone replacement therapy.

As always, nutritious diet, regular exercise, and continued involvement with your loved ones and community will help build resilience and ease the process of aging.

Breasts in Aging

With the loss of estrogen, the female breast tissue decreases in volume and becomes less full, losing mammary glands, fat, and tissue. Additionally, the connective tissue that lifts and supports the breast diminishes, causing the breasts to sag. Simultaneously, the nipple and surrounding tissue (*areola*) diminish. The areola may disappear, and the nipple may invert.[51]

The development of breast lumps is common in menopause, and usually is due to benign cysts. Naturally and appropriately, women should continue to self-examine their breasts at least monthly, as well as regular examination by their physician. Because we know breast cancer incidence increases with age, the recognition of any new breast lump should be examined by your physician or healthcare provider, often these days a physician's assistant or nurse practitioner. Furthermore, since self-breast examination is not 100% conclusive, the use of mammograms, ultrasounds, or MRIs of breast tissues should be discussed in depth with your primary care physician or gynecologist. These studies may be particularly helpful in women who have nodular breast tissue. The primary care physician or gynecologist can help you understand the risks and benefits of all these studies and help you arrive at examination and treatment options appropriate for your specific health concerns.[52]

Furthermore, many women wonder how long they need to continue to get mammograms and breast examinations. Most authorities recommend mammograms if there is at least 10 years of life expectancy. A 2014 review article in the Journal of the American Medical Association notes that age is the major risk factor for late-life breast cancer. We don't know the benefit of women over age 74, but the data does favor extending screening mammography to older women who are felt to have 5-10 years of life remaining. As for all women, benefits must be weighed with potential harms of continued screening over 10 years, which includes false-positives and over diagnosis which can lead to excessive or invasive testing.[53]

Bones, Muscles, and Joints in Aging

When we think of the aged, we often envision someone stooped over, white hair, wrinkled, and needing the assistance of a cane. Where a century or two ago, this posture might be attributable to someone in their 60s—assuming they even got to that age—this is a more likely the picture of octogenarians, nonagenarians, or centenarians. We may have more than 72,000 centenarians in the US alone; it may be one of the fastest growing portions of our population. That's good, I think.

The Skeletal System in Aging

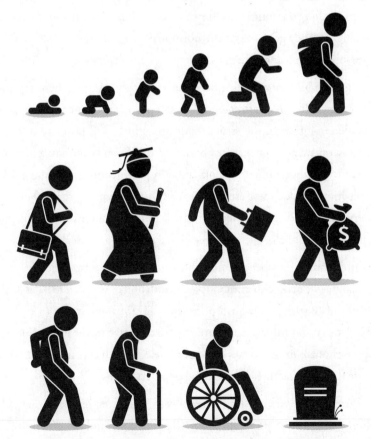

However, what accounts for the more typical bone, muscle, and joint characteristics that most of us experience as we age? Our skeleton allows for us to be erect, and yet flexible to accommodate a changing environment. Cartilage and synovial fluid between bones in the joint space keep bones from rubbing together and allow them to flex smoothly. Our muscles provide the power to move bones into proper alignment and motion.

Even though our brain remains the command center to coordinate movement, the proper health of our bones, muscles, and joints affect the quality of our motion. If any of these components lose their resilience, we may slow down or our motion may be less effective.[54]

So what actually changes in this erector set which holds us upright and propels us along our journey? Often, our bones may weaken, especially true in women as they go through the hormonal changes of menopause. Their bones lose calcium and other key minerals.

This introduces one of the most important topics in aging these days and that is the challenge of *osteoporosis*.[55] Osteoporosis is defined by low bone mass, deterioration of the structure of bone, increased porosity of bone, and subsequently, a higher risk of bone fracture. Frankly, most osteoporosis and associated bone fracture is observed in postmenopausal women, who are experiencing declining estrogen levels. This affects more than 10 million Americans. One dangerous feature of this illness is that it can be clinically silent—until a bone breaks with associated physical and fiscal sequelae.

Osteoporosis may become a major concern of our entire health system, especially as we make choices about our health dollar. We need to balance the cost of dual-energy X-ray absorptiometery (DXA bone scans) to evaluate bone density and initiate appropriate antiresorptive medications (like the bisphosphonate drugs) verses the cost of dealing with ever increasing costs to care for bone fractures in our aging population.

Current estimates are that osteoporosis is costing us more than $17 billion dollars (2005), 432,000 hospital admissions, and 2.5 million office visits. That pales in comparison to the fracture-related pain, disability, and diminishment of quality of life for our seniors.

It is important to note that osteoporosis is preventable and treatable.

Our current screening guidelines recommend screening women at least by age 65; but screening beyond that point is currently left to clinical judgment of the treating physicians. Occasionally, men and women below age 65 should also receive screening.

Although you can seek extensive guidelines for treatment of osteoporosis through your physician's office or off the Internet, here are just a few interventions for you to discuss with your doctors:

- Calcium and Vitamin D supplements: We all need adequate calcium and Vitamin D to maintain bone health and reduce risk of fractures. The recommendations are as follows: We should all be taking in 1,200 mg/day of calcium through diet or supplement. Adults age 50 or older should also take in 800-1,200 IU/day of Vitamin D (recommendations of the National Osteoporosis Foundation). There are slight variations from other health organizations, some of whom recommend less Vitamin D from 50 to 70 years of age, and others who offer slightly different recommendations for the amount of calcium.

- Our bones contain 99% of the calcium in our body, but when blood calcium lessens, our body turns to our bones for calcium. Vitamin D helps maintain serum calcium levels by enhancing small-intestinal absorption. We can get Vitamin D from sunlight exposure, fortified foods, egg yolks, saltwater fish, liver, and dietary supplements.[56]

- I know I sound like a broken record, but it is best to work directly with your primary care physician, your gynecologist, or your orthopedic surgeon to obtain the correct balance and dosing of these important products.

- There is also major benefit from weight-bearing exercise in maintaining bone strength. This will help posture, balance, agility, and prevent falls; however, exercise can increase the risk of fracture in some, so physician's guidance is necessary.

- Smoking and excessive alcohol also have detrimental effects on bone health. We cannot recommend any amount of smoking as helpful; however, it appears that only one drink per day for women and two or less per day for men might be allowable.

- Maintaining good vision and hearing, looking out for trip or fall hazards in the home, evaluating other medications that can add to imbalance, and evaluating neurological status may also benefit fracture-risk.

- There are a few so-called antiresorptive medications or selective estrogen-receptor modulators that have demonstrated benefit and can be discussed with your doctor.[57]

The shortening of our stature and the curvature of the spine come about as both the vertebrae (bones of our spine) collapse and the flexible, cushioning discs between the vertebrae lose fluid and elasticity. Not only do we begin to stoop over, but the compression of the vertebrae on each other and the arthritic spurs forming at the edges of the vertebrae may pinch nerves exiting the spinal column and produce substantial back and leg pain; this further limits mobility and exercise.

Further limiting our height, the arches of our feet flatten out. Although our long bones dwelling in our arms and legs might become thinner and more brittle, they generally don't shorten. This, however, makes us appear to have elongated extremities compared to our trunk.

Our joints become stiffer due to loss of cartilage and synovial fluid (the fluid keeping the joint lubricated), calcium may deposit along the joint edges, and inflammation may ensue, again limiting mobility. Even finger joints lose mobility and become painful, especially in women, and particularly in those who use their hands in repetitive, fine movement. One of the earliest joints to be affected by this degeneration is at the base of the thumb.

Muscle mass may lessen (atrophy) in men beginning in their twenties, and in women in their forties. Both bone and muscle strength can be helped by simple, modest weight lifting. As the nervous system ages, this affects the strength of muscles and muscle tone.

So what is the sum of all these gradual and subtle changes? We get shorter, less flexible, have less strength, and more painful movement. Our gait is slower, our stance is wider, our walking is unsteady, we feel more fatigued, and we have less get up and go!

Common Struggles in the Skeletal System

Women, in particular, develop *osteoporosis*, as we noted above. Bones break more easily in all parts of the body, especially the spine, again due to both hormonal changes and lessen mobility.

Because of muscle weakness we are less resilient and intolerant of activity and exercise. The muscle weakness also makes us lose balance, contributing to the easier fracture of brittle bones. Our automatic reflexes may lessen.

Some elderly also develop tremors, which often runs in family, and is also commonly associated with Parkinson's disease. Our muscles may just twitch on their own, referred to as *fasciculations.*

So how do we keep our mobility reasonably resilient? The good news here is we can make generally wise and helpful choices that can make a major difference to keep us mobile. Regular exercise is the key. Something as simple as using hand tools in the kitchen requiring our own power can make a difference. Choosing to walk rather than ride or drive, and rearranging our routine to encourage movement rather than a sedentary lifestyle are critical. Hide the remote, all you couch potatoes!

Get into an exercise class, but always check out your cardiovascular status with your healthcare provider, especially before starting a vigorous program.

We have already mentioned the importance of your nutrition, even at your advancing age.

Dietary calcium is also important for maintaining strong bones and teeth, and preserving blood, nerve, and other body tissue. Calcium helps us send nerve signals, helps our blood clot appropriately, helps us maintain a normal heartbeat, helps muscles contract and relax, and helps us release critical hormones and other chemicals.

We all know milk, yogurt, and cheese are good calcium sources, although we are aware of people who do not tolerate the proteins and sugars (lactose intolerance) in milk. Most pharmacies and most grocery stores have products to assist those with lactose intolerance and even have alternative products including lactose-free milk and other types of milk including coconut and almond milks. These may be far more acceptable to your gastrointestinal system if you're lactose intolerant. There are substantial concerns about the intolerance of milk proteins (whey and caseins) and milk sugar (lactose) and their effects on digestion and immunity in later life. A full discussion of this can be found in several wonderful articles on the subject including WebMD: What Is Lactose Intolerance, and WebMD: Milk Allergy: Products to Avoid, Foods with Milk in them and Tips.

Suffice it to say that dietary milk products supply calcium, phosphorus, and magnesium, and most milk is also fortified with vitamin D, although the sun remains our best source for this vitamin.

However, other foods contain good quantities of vitamin D, including nuts like almonds, sunflowers, and dried beans. Also green leafy vegetables like kale, broccoli, cabbage, and greens, and salmon and sardines with their soft, digestible bones, provide great sources of calcium. Anyone who is a good label-reader will recognize that calcium is also supplemented in numerous foods like orange juice, bread, and cereals.

If you wish to take further supplements, read the labels to make sure you are taking products with calcium citrate (more expensive but well-absorbed) or calcium carbonate (absorbed best if taken with food). Remember that there can be side effects from taking a large amount of calcium supplements, including kidney stones; consult your physician if you might have significant risk.

The recommendations for calcium to keep our bodies resilient are age-dependent but for adults ages 19-70 for men is 1,000 mg/day and for women pre-menopause 1,000 mg/day, bumped up to 1,200 mg/day post-menopause. Men can increase their calcium intake to 1,200 mg/day over age 70. Pregnant and/or nursing woman, if 14-18 years old, might want to increase calcium to 1,300 mg/day; and ages 19-50 may remain at 1,000 mg/day until menopause.

Just to help you understand what calcium you are getting in food, here's a helpful little list:

- 8 oz. glass of milk = 300 mg
- 6 oz. yogurt = 300 mg
- 1.5 oz. Swiss cheese = 300 mg
- ¼ cup of almonds = 100 mg
- One medium orange = 50 mg
- One medium baked sweet potato = 50 mg

Cardiac and Vascular Systems in Aging

The interplay of genetic and modifiable factors (diet, exercise, and other organ illnesses) is most pronounced in cardiovascular disease. Especially with the incidence of obesity in this country (beyond 35% of adults in 2017), the amount of cardiac, vascular, hypertensive, and stroke continues to run rampant. The good news is that we can make choices to alter the natural and aging course of this organ system by our health behavior.

Let's look at the cardiovascular system in detail, and then examine specific disorders that occur as we age. The heart has two sides; the right side receives blood coming back from its course in the body full of carbon dioxide and sends it to the lungs to expel the carbon dioxide and pick up oxygen. The left side of the heart sends oxygenated blood back out into the body. The heart is a marvelous complex of muscle, connective tissues, and a highly integrated nervous system.

The blood vessels gradually diminish in size from large arteries to small capillaries delivering blood products, nutrients, and oxygen. Blood is also brought by these vessels to the filtering systems of the liver and kidneys to dispose of waste.

Eventually, the capillaries pick up the waste from the body and return it through larger and larger vessels (veins) back to the heart.

Here are the major changes that occur in the heart in aging:

- The complex nervous system of the heart, controlled by a pacemaker center, can become fibrotic and take on fatty deposits. This can lead to altered rhythms in the heart or even a slow heart beat called *bradycardia*. The elderly can pass out from the slowed or altered rhythm.

- The wall of the heart may thicken and the heart may enlarge. Due to the thickening, the heart pump may actually become less efficient, pushing out less blood with each beat.

- Heart rhythms can change with aging. One can develop very erratic rhythms called *atrial fibrillation* or *arrhythmias* including extra beats from the lower chambers of the heart called *ventricular arrhythmias;* these can be dangerous.

- The pigment *lipofuscin* is often deposited in the heart and blood vessels with aging. The actual heart cells degenerate and the valves that control the direction of flow in the heart become thicker, stiffer, and less elastic, often producing heart murmurs.

Blood vessels are also affected in aging:

- Baroreceptors in the vessels that control the pressure within the vessels become less sensitive and may allow a person to pass out when standing from a sitting or lying position. This happens because less blood goes up to the brain.

- As capillary walls thicken, nutrients and wastes are less effectively exchanged.

- There is a thickening and hardening of the great vessel coming from the heart, the aorta, and this raises blood pressure and makes the heart work harder, thicken, and stiffen. This great vessel may also balloon (aneurysm) or rupture.[58]

Finally, the blood itself may also change with aging:

- With aging, the total volume of blood decreases and the blood has less fluid in it.

- The speed with which the bone marrow reproduces and replenishes blood cells decreases.

- Although white blood cells stay about the same in number, those specifically prepared to fight infection (neutrophils) do decrease in number. We are less able to fight invaders like bacteria.

To summarize, as we age our heart becomes a less effective pump. It is less resilient to challenges like infection, emotional stress, exercise, injuries, and certain types of medicines.

Complicating these many natural aging changes in the heart, vessels, and blood, a variety of additional ailments can complicate the aging heart:

- *Atherosclerosis*, a hardening of arteries due to the buildup of inflammation and fatty deposits, can narrow and even block arteries and flow. When this occurs within the blood vessels of the heart, we may experience a heart attack or *myocardial infarction* (MI).

- Preceding a heart attack, we may have warning symptoms telling us blood flow to the heart is being limited; this may be in the form of chest pain or *angina,* shortness of breath, especially with exertion.

- If the heart muscle has been significantly damaged due to reduced blood flow or an infarction, often with resulting heart scar tissue, we may experience *congestive heart failure* (CHF).

- Abnormal rhythms of the heart may occur with aging, but also due to medications, atherosclerosis, or cardia nerve dysfunction.

- We may develop low blood count or *anemia* from illnesses that block production in the bone marrow, chronic infections or medications, or that lead to increased loss of blood from gastrointestinal bleeding.

- Blood pressure medicine needs to be adjusted to maintain appropriate pressure in the cardiovascular system. Our new parameters for blood pressure suggest that we want to keep our pressure in the 120/80 range. Just as we fully understand the importance of treating blood pressure elevation and the benefits of such care, it is also worth noting that in elderly patients, we need to be careful not to *over treat* blood pressure. To much medication can lead to *hypotension* (low or inadequate blood pressure) as well as *orthostatic hypotension*, where the blood pressure suddenly drops upon rising from a sitting or lying position. Orthostatic hypotension can cause fainting and falls.[59]

- Heart valves may leak (aortic or mitral regurgitation) or become thickened and narrow (aortic or mitral stenosis) all leading to ineffective pumping.

- If blood flow to the brain is disrupted, we can suffer a transient ischemic attack (TIA) or stroke.

As if these problems were not enough, we can also develop blood clots in arteries or in deep veins (thrombosis), inflammation in the veins (thrombophlebitis), varicose veins, narrowing in the arteries of the legs due to atherosclerosis and causing leg pain with exertion (claudication), and ballooning of the arteries due to wall weakness and injury (aneurysms). Sudden blowouts or ruptures of aneurysms are highly likely to cause death.

How can we add resilience and wellness to our cardiovascular complex? There is an unquestionable genetic component to heart and vessel disease as we know many families where disorders in this system lead to great disability and early death. The way our bodies handle fat and waste, glucose, and salt, and balance pressure in the system, plus various structural problems in the heart muscle, valves, and wiring all have familial factors.

However, whether our family has a propensity for heart disease or not, there are a plethora of healthy behavioral habits we can employ to preserve and improve this system.

- **Dietary choices:** Heart-healthy diets limit saturated fats and cholesterol. Rather than animal, particularly red meat fats, consume fats based in vegetables, nuts, fish like salmon, and legumes. You should probably consume red meat in small quantity (5-6 oz.) once per week; if you love meat protein consider fish two times per week.

Taking the approach of a *plant-slant* to your diet—that is consuming 90% of your diet as fruits, veggies, and whole grain products, which will substantially help to control *obesity, diabetes,* and *hypertension,* all major factors in the development of cardiovascular disease.[60]

- **Movement:** Note here I am emphasizing the term *movement* rather than *exercise.* Exercise can be one of the key components of your *movement* program. The American Heart Association tells us for good heart health we should be exercising approximately 150 minutes per week. Another way to quantify that is five 30-minutes exercise sessions per week. This exercise should be enough to get our target heart rate above roughly 65% of our maximum rate for age and there are many charts that can quantify that for you.

However, I am really stressing here the importance of general movement, especially as we age. I'm talking about making simple changes in our daily behavior, like walking rather than riding, taking stairs rather than elevators or escalators, and using hand-operated cooking utensils rather than electric products. Add increased movement to the basic tasks of living.

If you have not been an *exerciser* in the past, see your healthcare provider first to get a baseline status on the old ticker. If your physician believes you're in adequate shape to begin, start slowly with a walking and stretching program. Slowly add some modest weight lifting. Consider a gym membership where you will have guidance and encouraging support. Strongly consider a good pair of walking or running shoes with good arch support and heel cushion.

Be aware that exercise is a terrific stress-reducer. It is a wonderful way to begin your day or add a period of time at midday or in the late afternoon to clear the body, mind, and spirit of the toxins of stress.

There is substantial interest in wearable monitoring devices for aging people to make sure that they are obtaining enough physical activity to keep them autonomous, independent, and physical functioning with efficiency and with the avoidance of limitations in their mobility.

There are a number of important activity behaviors that would be helpful to monitor: physical activity and sedentary behavior, posture detection and transition times, daily activity classification, energy expenditure, fatigue detection, detection and prediction of falling events, gait analysis and balance, tremor and freezing events, sleep analysis, and location-awareness. Wearable wrist monitors, GPS units, wearable cameras, and wireless communication technologies are all being developed to accomplish these tasks at a cost-effective manner. Advanced prototypical activity trackers, advanced algorithms for activity, posture, falling, gait, and balance analysis are all in various stages of development and implementation. Stay tuned![61]

- **Smoking:** STOP. Stop immediately. There is overwhelming evidence of the damage smoking does to your heart, lungs, skin, and bladder among other organs. There is also excellent evidence that cessation of smoking has immediate and undoubted long-term benefits. Please stop, and again, see your healthcare provider for products and programs to assist you in this most important change in health behavior.

- **Doctor:** See the doctor regularly. Make heart screening a part of a regular visit to your healthcare provider, especially if you have a previous history of heart or lung disease or these run in your family. This should include an assessment of risk factors, including a check of your blood pressure, lipids, glucose, and kidney function. If you have been a smoker, and especially if you are a male between 65 and 75, you should periodically be assessed for the development of an aneurysm in the great arteries leading from the heart, particularly the aorta.

Lungs in Aging

The lungs have two purposes: getting oxygen (O2) *in* from the air and get carbon dioxide (CO2) from our metabolism *out*. Our body needs oxygen to work properly and it needs to dispose of carbon dioxide as a byproduct of using that oxygen so that resilience and homeostasis can be reestablished.

Air comes in through the mouth and nose when we inhale and is transported through the airway into smaller and smaller tubes to the small cavities or sacs in lung tissue that are surrounded by tiny blood vessels. Oxygen enters the bloodstream at this interface and carbon dioxide is removed from the blood at this same place and expelled as we exhale.

In aging, there are a variety of organ systems and tissues that interact and each influences the other. Let us look at several systems and examine their effect on oxygen and carbon dioxide exchange in aging.[62]

Bones and muscles of the chest and spine: Because of bony thinning and bending, the ribcage may lose its shape, so that you cannot inhale and exhale as efficiently. The muscular diaphragm, or large flat muscle between the lung cavity and the abdominal cavity may weaken; again inhalation and exhalation are diminished. We can develop fatigue and shortness of breath just because we are not getting adequate O2 or are retaining CO2. Also, the curvature of the spine in aging may diminish ability to inhale adequately or exhale completely.

Lung tissue: The tissue making up the respiratory tree deteriorates in aging. The tiny lung sacs become less elastic, and the muscles between the ribs and lining the airways become weaker. Again, we are unable to exchange O2 and CO2 efficiently.[63]

Respiratory nervous innervation: Breathing is under the control of areas in the brain. If the brain deteriorates, it may well affect breathing. Furthermore, the nerves in your airways that trigger the coughing reflex may diminish, and then you are unable to expel toxic particles or infectious agents like bacteria.[64]

Respiratory immune system: As your immunity weakens, you are less able to mount a defense to toxins and infection. If you are exposed to smoke or other particulate irritants, you are less able to recover. You are less resilient.

Finally, as our respiratory system weakens we are more likely to develop pneumonia or bronchitis. This lessens the O2 supply to all tissues and affects their function. We can develop abnormal breathing patterns, such as sleep apnea where we actually stop breathing for a prolonged period of time with acute and chronic trauma to our brain, heart, and nervous system.[65]

What can we do to preserve, restore, and strengthen resilience in the respiratory tree?

- Stop smoking. Smoking injures the lung and heart tissue and speeds deterioration of the lungs.

- Exercise regularly. This strengthens lung muscle and builds breathing capacity.

- Move, move, move, especially after lying down and particularly after surgical procedures.

- Limit the amount of products that cause allergic and respiratory ailments like asthma, bronchitis, and allergic rhinitis by modifying your environment, especially in your home.[66] Energy efficiency in our homes (where we spend much of our time as we age) has made our homes closed environments with a higher potential for exposure to contaminants. Paying attention to pet exposure, changing bedding frequently and following bedding instructions for cleaning, using air purification systems, and pest management can all pay substantial dividends in controlling air within the home. Of course, the cessation of smoking in the home to avoid second-hand smoke exposure is a keystone of care.

Sleep in Aging

Sleep is a critical function for humans at all ages and sleep affords us resiliency in multiple aspects of our body, mind, and, I would suggest, our spirit. Sleep helps restore function to most organ systems. It particularly helps refresh and reorganize the brain. Let us look at what transpires as we sleep to better understand the effects of aging.

Sleep has two core components: First, a period of dreamlessness both in light and deep sleep. Second, we experience periods of active dreaming call REM (rapid eye movement) sleep. We sleep in cycles between dreaming and non-dreaming and several cycles occur each night.[67]

As we age, we generally have a harder time falling asleep; we awaken more frequently during sleep; and we arise earlier in the morning. The total sleep time remains roughly the same (between 5.5 and 8 hours) for most of us. There are several excellent and recent studies that suggest all of us should try to have 7-8 hours of sleep nightly, no matter our age.

The transition time between sleep and wake happens more quickly with aging, making us feel we are not experiencing deep or good sleep. Less time is spent in deep dreamless sleep. Additionally, there are many other factors that disrupt sleep as we age including having to get up to urinate, pain of arthritis and other illnesses, and anxiety and depression. Many older people will awaken 3-4 times every night, even if they spend more total time in bed.

Trouble sleeping is an extremely aggravating situation and can lead to auto accidents, irritability, and depression. Insomnia, if progressive, can lead to mental changes including substantial confusion. Depression may result from insomnia, or may be at the core of the underlying sleep abnormality. A thorough evaluation and mental health history are critical to successful therapy.

Although insomnia is the most common sleep problem for elderly folks, additional disorders such as sleep apnea, restless leg syndrome, narcolepsy (sudden falling asleep in the course of natural activity), and hypersomnia also increase with age.[68]

There is also a growing body of evidence that insomnia may well be a risk factor for the development of Alzheimer's disease and that getting a good night of sleep may assist us in preventing cognitive (thinking) impairment.[69]

What can we do to improve sleep as we age?

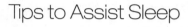

Tips to Assist Sleep

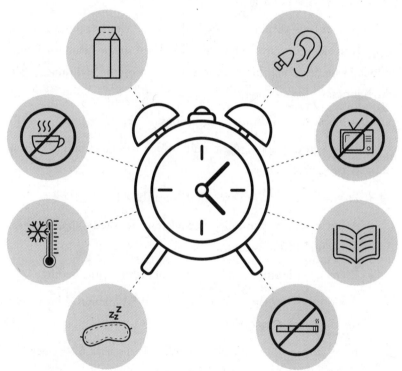

Sadly, a common quick fix in our society is sedation and sleeping medications, particularly requiring a prescription. As often as possible, these should be avoided.

Elderly react differently to medications, particularly sedative drugs, than younger people. It is important to consult your healthcare provider, who is familiar with your medical conditions and your other medications, before beginning any sleeping drugs.

If depression is an issue for you, an antidepressant might be more beneficial than sedation medications. Perhaps a trial with a mild antihistamine or melatonin (a hormone naturally made by the pineal gland but also available as an over-the-counter medication) would help, as long as your other medications won't interfere. Generally, we try to limit use of antihistamines in the elderly because of other potential effects on the genitourinary system or heart.

The use of any sleeping sedatives should be closely monitored and probably avoided on any long-term basis. Used in excess or for longer periods, these drugs may build up to toxic levels causing delirium or falls with injuries.

A few simple non-medication suggestions may help:

- Have a small glass of warm milk, which has a naturally occurring sedative protein in it.
- Have a light snack, not excessively sugar-based.
- Avoid stimulants like coffee, chocolate, caffeinated sodas, or tea for 3-4 hours prior to bedtime.
- Exercise in the afternoon but not immediately before bedtime.
- Avoid excessive naps; try to limit to 20-30 minutes so as to not interfere with sleep cycles.
- Keep your room temperature cool, perhaps near 62-65 degrees, which helps simulate a hibernating state.
- Keep your room dark or utilize a sleeping mask.
- Keep your room quiet or utilize earplugs.
- Avoid excessively stimulating TV shows immediately before bed.
- Make reading enjoyable rather than tedious.
- Try to go to bed and wake up at roughly the same times daily; get into a discipline.

- Avoid tobacco products and vaporizing smoking agents.

- Double-check with your health provider to make sure you are not on other medications that alter sleep.

- Although many people find they fall asleep better with a small glass of wine, often alcohol will make you awaken frequently or earlier during the night.

- If it takes you longer than 20 minutes to fall asleep, get up and move to another room to do light reading or listen to music. If you then are unsuccessful at falling asleep, give it another try before trying other methods.[70]

Nervous System in Aging

Having looked at these many organ systems that make up the human body and what happens to them in aging, we are about to move to an examination of our cognition, our thinking, processing, emotions, and memory. Since we now understand that much of this activity flows within our brain and nervous system and, possibly, interactions with what we might call our ethereal spiritual selves, let's move a discussion of our central and peripheral nervous system into Chapter Five: Our Minds as We Age.

CHAPTER 5

OUR MINDS AS WE AGE—KEEPING AND SHINING AT LEAST MOST OF OUR MARBLES

When we stop to ponder the process of aging, I suspect most of us are distressed about the possibilities and reality of losing our memories and our abilities to be attentive, to perceive, and communicate effectively, especially with loved ones. We may also fear the loss of value that our experience and intellect might hold for the tribe with whom we live and serve. Quite simply, we are afraid of "losing our marbles." As physical changes and diminished capacities may limit our independence, our mental prowess and acuity may dramatically isolate us from the highly desired interactions with others that we know adds immeasurably to the quality of our lives.

Therefore I want to tie this chapter into the previous discussion of our changing physical selves by first examining the anatomy and function of our central and peripheral nervous system with age. Then we will look at the heterogeneous (variable, diverse) cognitive capabilities we see in our aging population as that realization is most pertinent to this discussion.

The Nervous System Itself

The brain and nervous system are the central control panel and connective wiring for your body; additionally, they regulate your thoughts and memories, attentiveness, movement, and senses. This communication network also modulates other organs like your heart and gastrointestinal tract.

Nerves are the interstate highways and country roads connecting your brain with all parts of the body, and extend out from a long, main spinal cord that runs inside of your vertebrae called the spinal column.

As you age, your nervous system gradually loses function and capacity by getting smaller (atrophying) and losing nerve cells themselves and the supporting cells (glial cells) around them. Messages are passed more slowly and waste accumulates in the neural tissue as cells break down. Plaques and nerve tangles begin to accumulate in brain tissue, particularly in those suffering from Alzheimer's. Additionally, lipofuscin, a fatty brown pigment, also gathers in the nerve tissue. With the breakdown of nerve cells comes a diminishment of senses, reflexes, and movement.[71]

The speed of thought and the storage of memory also diminish in aging, but this varies widely in individuals. Some loss of thought capacity is normal with aging, but when this becomes excessive and memory loss pronounced, we might be dealing with actual diseases like *dementia* or *Alzheimer's*. The two most common forms of dementia are cerebrovascular dementia (due to atherosclerotic build-up and narrowing) and Alzheimer's. Our current evidence is that Alzheimer's, at least, is related to the buildup of lipofuscin, plaques, and nerve tangles in the brain.[72]

Another disorder associated with sudden confusion is called *delirium*. More often concurrent medical illnesses such as acute or chronic infections or medications likely are the source of delirium[73] and, frankly, anything that leads to loss of hydration can make the aging individual more susceptible to delirium.

Uncontrolled diabetes can also lead to disorders of thought and memory.

If you notice sudden thought, behavior, or memory change in yourself or loved ones, seek attention from your healthcare provider as soon as possible. The change from your baseline mentation is important and a potential warning sign of other physical or cognitive illnesses.

Thinking in Aging

Much of the function of the nervous system and brain is involved in what we call *thinking*. We have just examined what happens to the brain and nervous system as we age from a structural and functional standpoint. What about this rather unique collection of *thinking processes* that seem to be so highly developed in humans?

The medical term we apply to the daily activity of thinking is *cognition*. To age successfully, we probably need a level of cognition that allows us to interact with our environment, including our effective and appropriate relational interactions within and outside of ourselves. Cognition allows us to perceive, understand, and then respond to our environment. Our ability to feed, dress, bathe, and use the toilet are all highly dependent on our cognitive ability and resilience. Furthermore, our effectiveness in interacting with those around us is critical to aging well.

Cognition *does* change with age, and it is important to note that there are significant physical, behavioral, and social factors that influence our cognition with time. There is strong evidence to support effective interventions that may optimize our cognition as we grow older. We will look at a few of these.

We know that many medical conditions and medications can adversely affect our thinking. On the other hand, defective thinking with age can cause us to incorrectly understand our physicians' instructions, particularly regarding preventive health strategies.

Cognition includes a variety of mental functions including general intellect, language, memory, attention, visuospatial skills, visual and auditory perception, and problem solving. But as we consider multiple interrelated functions, just how do we define successful cognitive aging?

Here are a few of the definitions of aging with effective maintenance of cognition:

- There are batteries of cognitive tests given to aging folks, and scoring above the mean can be one definition of successful aging.[74]

- Stability over time and maintaining intact cognitive skills could be another definition.

- An alternative definition is simply people who have *not* had to experience minimal interruption of activities of daily living from a cognitive standpoint. This definition implies that success means a person can interact with their environment and adapt, accommodate, and adjust to age-related changes.[75] In a sense, this signifies a *resilient* cognition.

The later definition is probably most meaningful to most of us interested in cognition in aging. I suspect that includes you.

So what is actually known about the factors that influence cognition with age, particularly what we would label intelligence, and what factors are probably not as important or influential on our thinking as we get older?

Cognition appears to contain two categories of intelligence:

- Crystallized intelligence: learned, familiar skills we gather through both education and practice. Included in this category are knowledge of facts and our vocabulary; both increase quickly in our youth and then stabilize or gradually improve with age. Our verbal ability remains fairly constant. Procedural memory such as riding a bike or driving a car may be maintained since they are overlearned skills.

- Fluid intelligence: non-verbal reasoning, motor skills, and problem-solving abilities that change as we age. Fluid intelligence improves throughout childhood and adolescence, gradually declines in adulthood, but rapidly declines in old age. The loss of nerve volume, connections, and increased rates of other illnesses and injuries may have cumulative effects.[76]

Intelligence in Aging

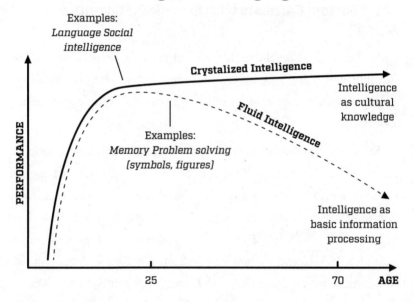

With cognitive features that remain stable, change, or deteriorate with age it should be noted that there is *immense variation* between specific individuals. Genetic differences, concomitant diseases, socioeconomic differences, and levels of intellectual and environmental stimulation, as well as personality may all influence cognitive aging. These widely varying differences have led to a newer catchphrase particularly pertinent to cognition called "heterogeneity of aging."[77] A significant factor to consider in the wide variations in cognitive success or deterioration in aging is that with time we become more different because we simply have had more time to get this way! So notes Dr. David Carr, aforementioned professor of geriatric medicine and neurology at the Washington University School of Medicine in St. Louis, and a leading expert on aging.

Furthermore, with the help of aids, social support, technological assistance, and general good physical activity, many people who do experience declining cognition can still live successfully and compensate for age-related losses.

What Factors Correlate with Successful Cognitive Aging?

Undoubtedly there are physical, psychological, and social/cultural factors that influence cognition with age. Once again, there are broad differences among people in cognitive function in aging, as multiple studies have shown.

Most evidence reveals that overall intellectual function declines in the oldest individuals studied (80s-100s), but everyday problem solving and function remain relatively intact, in the absence of neurodegenerative disease (Alzheimer's, dementia, stroke). One strong predictor of cognition in later life is the level of *educational achievement*. Those with higher educational levels tend to show less intellectual decline with age and tend to demonstrate less dementia or Alzheimer's.[78, 79, 80] It is unclear whether this is due to developing increased reserve or whether higher education is proxy for additional factors that benefit brain health such as an active and healthy lifestyle.

Lack of physical activity, as well as illnesses that also limit physical activity such as cardiac disease, or the use of tobacco and alcohol all appear to predict worse cognitive functioning in aging. In particular, cardiovascular disease and related hospitalizations tend to highly affect cognition. Conversely, consistent exercise, good pulmonary capacity, and good cardiovascular health all positively influence cognition.[81]

What about our emotional wellness and ability to handle stress? We understand that depression and anxiety appear to negatively impact cognitive health and these emotions occur more frequently in people with diminished intellectual health. In general, it is well-established that with old age, there is an increase in both anxiety and depression. At times, the cognitive reductions observed with depression can be mistaken for dementia, sometimes referred to as "pseudodementia." Factors that can separate out pseudodementia from true dementia include classic symptoms of depression including apathy, loss of motivation/interest, lack of enjoyment and disruptions of sleep and appetite.[82] Yet the differences between true dementia and pseudodementia remain a significant diagnostic dilemma for physicians providing care to these individuals.

Further, one's belief that one can positively influence a desired outcome by one's personal behavior highly correlates with better cognition with age. When people feel valued, purposed, feel "worth their salt" to their family or their community, they engage in life and in relationships.

What Type of Interventions Help Our Thinking as We Age?

The media is filled with articles and advertisement urging us to partake in activities that stimulate our memory. Are these efforts worthwhile?

Although the studies vary as to which specific memory training programs consistently produce the best results, there appears to be consensus that memory training does help cognition in aging. Memory loss can be substantially sobering.[83]

Nonetheless, there is hope![84]

Of particular interest are memory techniques that pair places or objects in a familiar room in your home with items you might want to remember to purchase at a grocery store. You are asked to visually associate the grocery item with another familiar object. This appears to enhance memory.[85]

Another technique for helping remember the names of people, for example, involves pairing the person's name with a particular physical characteristic: Michael has a mustache; Betty has blonde hair, and so forth. This is called "pretraining" and helps prepare a person for mnemonic memory techniques. These techniques all seem to help "episodic memory" where we are trying to recall peoples' names, or remember appointments, or special dates. Most studies show that this sort of training is maintained for a prolonged number of years, not just short term, but that is does generally decline slowly with age.

Episodic memory training serves best for remembering the specific items, names, circumstances that the memory training is specifically targeting. However, there is no evidence that episodic memory training enhances all memory for future important targets, like future appointments. There may be great value in just helping convince you that you do have some control on intellectual factors as you age, such as memory, through these proactive resilience techniques; you may well lessen anxiety.[86, 87]

General Lifestyle Strategies to Preserve Cognition in Aging

We have previously emphasized the importance of repeated physical exercise and movement for all health, but it applies equally to preserving intellectual function, dealing with stress and anxiety, and helping prevent depression.

Continuing education and *lifelong learning* also appear to improve cognition in aging.

There is much interest in several supplemental medications that appear to be helpful. Estrogen supplements in older women appear to help reasoning, concept formation, and verbal memory, but have *not* been proven effective. So at this time caution needs to be exercised before consistently prescribing estrogen to all aging women, and the potential risks associated with other concomitant illnesses always must be taken into account by the prescribing physician.[88, 89, 90]

What Risk Factors Impair Cognition with Age?

Dementia

We've covered topics that can preserve and improve cognition, but let us return to a more in depth discussion of factors that impair our thought processes with aging. When we think of impaired cognition, we think of *dementia*, and most often the first intellectual loss we think of with dementia includes the loss of memory. However, to really make a diagnosis of dementia requires additional impairment in cognitive activities like loss of language or motor dexterity, diminished judgment, planning, abstract reasoning, attention, visuospatial skill, and impaired occupational, social, or common activities of daily living.

Sadly, dementia and related illnesses are increasingly common in the U.S. Perhaps as many as 3-7 million Americans suffer from these types of cognitive dysfunction. As alluded to earlier, Alzheimer's and vascular dementia (due to hardening of the arteries to and in the brain) account for about 75% of the cases. But other diagnosis like dementia due to alcoholism, Parkinson's disease or Lewy body disease, and frontal lobe dementia are also common.

Any illnesses that affect the vascular system, like diabetes, stroke, hypertension, elevated cholesterol and other lipids, and, of course, smoking, all contribute to worsening dementia in aging.

Alzheimer's

Alzheimer's affects about 5% of adults older than 65, and 20% to 50% of adults older than 80—no small number. Research in Alzheimer's has been aggressive with such a high penetrance in our society, and hope lies in finding genetic and environmental factors that we can modify. An additional area of research has focused on familial genetics in Alzheimer's patients; there is promising data showing gene mutations on several chromosomes that appear to be strongly related in certain families with high incidence of Alzheimer's. Furthermore, we see some genetic factors that also cause coronary artery disease associated with Alzheimer's. Even diabetes mellitus appears to increase dementia threefold in midlife.[91, 92]

Miscellaneous Causes of Dementia

Several environmental factors like antioxidants and estrogens are being studied because they might have preventative effects on dementia. Vitamin E also has received some attention in recent studies. The power of these supplements most likely contributes to a multifaceted and complex prevention rather than a single agent helping stop the progression of dementia.[93]

What Treatment Options Are Available Right Now for Alzheimer's and to Help Prevent Cognitive Decline in General Thinking and Processing?

Although most dementia, like Alzheimer's, does not generally completely reverse with treatment, it is always worth examining a person for potentially reversible illnesses like hypothyroidism and B12 deficiency, which can be helped dramatically with therapy.

There is a growing interest in an antibody associated with a very rare form of cognitive impairment sometimes referred to as "brain on fire." This condition involves the body creating antibodies against a brain receptor called NMDA (N-Methl-D-aspartic acid).[94]

At present, for Alzheimer's therapy, we have two classes of drugs: the cholinesterase inhibitors (donepezil, revastigmine, galantamine) and NMDA [N-Methyl-D-aspartic acid] antagonists (memantine). In general, these medications have been shown to increase the time dementia patients can be on their own (prior to assisted living). These drugs typically only help those with mild and moderate dementia and are not effective for severe dementia. Even if patients have a positive response to medications, a progressive neurodegenerative disease such as Alzheimer's disease will cause further decline. These drugs are not thought to be disease-modifying agents; in other words, they don't cure or stop the progression of the underlying disease itself.

Two other supplements, Vitamin E and selegiline (Emsam, Zelapar, Eldepryl), although originally showing promise in slowing progression of Alzheimer's in some patients,[95] actually have limited evidence and are now rarely recommended.

In summary, for general cognition, six major factors seem to be associated with the impairment of cognitive function with aging:

- Lower educational level[96]
- Poor physical health and physical activity[97]
- Poor emotional wellbeing, including anxiety, depression, and perceived ability to be not able to do things in order to solve challenges[98]
- Minimal social engagement[99]
- Poor diet[100]
- Risk factors for atherosclerosis[101]

The definitive causes of dementia and Alzheimer's disorders are largely still unknown. However, the most consistent predictor of dementia is age itself. Genetic predisposition is also a significant predictor. Social engagement and a stable social environment are also being studied as having positive influences on dementia. Finally, we do have medications and behavioral adjustment programs that seem to offer some modest relief to the unrelenting deterioration in cognition of dementia disorders.

We do have hope, through aggressive research and study, public concern, and advocacy for patients and their families suffering from cognitive dysfunction with aging.

Where Do We Go from Here?

Are there things that we can do to add resilience to our mental health and memory even if we are not dealing directly with dementia or Alzheimer's?

There are aspects of enhancing brain fitness that we do have good scientific evidence to support. We touched on the importance of exercise and movement, but we do know that physical exercise stimulates the growth of brain size and intra-brain connections. Increased blood flow may be a significant factor in this growth.

For most of us, simple brain-exercise measures and "brain games" such as playing mind-stimulating games like cards or computer programs, looking at old photographs and recalling people, places, and circumstances, reading, crossword puzzles, and engaging in conversation will all benefit mental resilience. As we mentioned, memory training improves function and the brain becomes more efficient; a particularly interesting study of surgeons demonstrates better decision-making and hand-eye coordination. Friends, make sure your surgeon plays Game Boy or Dr. Mario before he/ she grabs the scalpel.

There are also an increasing number of brain-games or brain-stimulating electronic programs. Anecdotally, many people report improvement in memory and brain computation function. Most scientific researchers have yet to develop accurate ways to study and measure the effect of these games on the brain. In fact there is a growing body of evidence that suggests brain games are not effective for most types of cognition.[102] Programs like Lumosity and other cognitive games must await further study. I would suggest these brain-stimulation programs are probably not detrimental, and, therefore, if you enjoy them, play away.

Attention should also focus on the importance of socialization and social networks to benefit cognition. We may reference back to the Blue Zone observations and how having small groups of close-knit friends seems to maintain intellectual acuity and the feeling of being needed and contributing to community life. Several newer studies support this observation.[103, 104]

Working on a computer, we also understand, increases brain efficiency and assists peripheral vision, no matter at what age we start utilizing this device.

Regarding memory, two of the leading experts on brain fitness, Dr. Gary Small and his wife, Gigi Vorgan, describe a simple memory strategy that has substantial benefit. They call it *Look, Snap, Connect*. When remembering a person, situation, or setting that is important to you, use the following process:[105, 106]

- *Look*: Focus on what is before you. Concentrate on the person or circumstance at hand. Use tunnel vision to focus on that memory subject.

- *Snap*: Take a mental snap-shot of your subject.

- *Connect*: Make a mental connection of the subject with another name or circumstance, which may help you recall the subject. For example, if you meet somehow whose name is Chuck, connect his name with something else, like chuck-wagon. Or, if you meet a person named Sue, and they happen to be a lawyer, there's an easy memory-connect: sue-Sue.

If you do this repeatedly, it will become second nature.

I cannot understate the importance of regular physical activity and good nutrition that will assist brain resiliency by increasing blood flow and reducing cell death in the nervous tissues. Diet and exercise decrease the potential damage from hypertension, hyperlipidemia, obesity, and diabetes, all major risk factors for disease in the aging brain.

Once again, successful intellectual function/cognition with age means that a person can interact with other persons and with a changing environment and adapt to those age-related changes. More simply stated, successful older adults have a minimal interruption of their usual level of daily function.

So, successful cognition in aging requires focus on a wide cadre of intellectual skills including memory, language, complex problem-solving, visual-spatial skills, attention, personality, and general intellectual ability. What make these studies on cognition particularly challenging are the vast individual variations that occur across the population. Furthermore, it may be only one or two of these intellectual functions that decline, while others remain well in a given individual. Nonetheless, we remain strongly hopeful of breakthroughs in the numerous public and private research studies in process as we advance through the 21st century. Stay tuned for the exciting news on the horizon.

CHAPTER 6

THE SOUL AND SPIRIT IN AGING—CONSTANT OR WAXING AND WANING?

" Now I lay me down to sleep,

I pray the Lord my *soul* to keep,

If I should die before I wake,

I pray the Lord my *soul* to take.

Amen."

Recently, I came across a couple of additional lines that I cherish:

"And if in morning light I wake,

Show me the path of love to take."

You might have knelt at the bedside and recited this children's prayer in the presence of your parents as did I, or again with your young ones. The words of this prayer succinctly encompass the core of *soul-ness* in each one of us. They portray the simple faith of childhood, but powerfully linger especially in an aging body, mind, and spirit. The words also encompass the core of *soul-ness* as I am defining it throughout the book: the capacity to *fear, love,* and *trust* God.

Just as with our physical bodies and minds, change and faltering may exist within the *soul* as well. As Christians, we know and believe that we have a spiritual aspect to our being. We each have a soul in which the spiritual essence of who we are in Christ resides. Our souls are what Christ came to save, and our souls are where faith and hope in him are found. God is faithful to the relationship restored in God's creatures and creation through Christ's sacrifice. God does not falter or change. In Christ, we are assured of God's unconditional, unalterable *love.*

But doubt and uncertainty about the nature of our souls from our human perspective can creep in, especially as we grow older, and particularly in light of a deteriorating body or a confused and wandering mind. Additionally, we may find ourselves asking, "What exactly happens to me when I die?" We see and know that our physical bodies cease operating and will turn to dust, but what about our souls?

Much remains, and will remain, an enigma until we meet our Creator face to face and until God brings complete healing to a fallen, disordered, and diseased creation. But what we know to be true from Scripture is that the *soul* is mysterious and integral to being human and that it is a precious gift to each of us from a loving, continuously engaged, trustworthy Creator.

The Soul Defined

In Genesis 2:7, we read, *"Then the Lord God formed a man from the <u>dust of the ground</u> and breathed into his nostrils the <u>breath of life,</u> and the man <u>became a living being (soul).</u>"* The Creator God forms humankind not only out of created material elements, but also *makes* the material a living being, a whole, a soul, by placing God's spirit or breath within it. It is our *soul* that flows from a relational Being, God. Our God is a relational God, a God who loves us and wants to be with us.

Therefore, we might better say that we do not have a soul, we *are* a soul.

But though we were made in God's image and were meant to live in harmony with our God, when sin entered the world that perfect unity was lost; God sought to reestablish the relationship with us, with our souls. God did that through Jesus, God's Son, who died to redeem our souls from this horrid separation, from the clench of death.

Furthermore, the human creature may be made in the *image of God* (as suggested in Chapter One—the capacity to *fear, love,* and *trust*), but is *not* God. That "capacity to *love*" appears to be a special, highly significant, shared, relational nature of the human creature and the Creator. The rest of God's creation, and that would include *lesser animals,* relates to God as *Creator* and *Sustainer,* and man as their *steward* (Genesis 1:26-27), but, scripturally, does not appear to share with man or God the *love-centered image* of God.

So God and humankind share a relationship distinct from other animals. Yet man and animals also share a relationship distinct from God; neither humankind, nor animals, nor anything else in creation are immune to the effects of *sin.* Both humans and animals have physical natures susceptible to *sin.*

There is a most important second aspect of *love* as a part of the soul of a human, and that is the soul's *assurance of being loved* by the Creator. (Matthew 10:30-31 and John 3:16) I suspect, at the root of most of the distress and emotional ills we face as humans, the *doubting that we are loved* turns out to be the very seed of our troubles. That seed of doubt is sin.

Now there is much speculation on how this redemption of our souls will happen when we die; we will never truly know the exact details this side of heaven. What we do know for sure as Christians is that at death, we will be with God, joined with God in inconceivable joy, eternally. What we can know without question (because we are told so in God's Word) is that God is loving, so loving that God sent Christ from the splendor of heaven into the pain of earth, and even into the depths of hell, in our place so that we could be with the Creator into eternity. God has the plan; God has the vision; God provides the pathway in Jesus. Jesus is preparing the way and the destiny (John 14:2-4), even as we are aging.

As Paul tells us in 1 Thessalonians 5:23:

"May God himself, the God of peace, sanctify you through and through. May your whole spirit, soul, and body be kept blameless at the coming of our Lord Jesus Christ."

That's good enough for me, and I pray through Jesus that it is for you.

Thoughts on the Soul

Some of you may have more in depth questions about traditional and contemporary writings on soul-topics such as:

- When is the soul created?
- Why is the soul created?
- Perspectives on Purgatory and Grace?
- Is the soul uniquely human?
- Is the soul asleep in death?
- What is the soul in the doctrine of law and gospel?
- Does the soul age? The doctrines of passive and active righteousness.

These are important and interestingly challenging topics and I would invite you to visit the appendix for discussion.

Care of the Soul in Aging

Until that time when our souls are reunited with God in heaven, how should we care for our souls as we age?

Of course, you might think, is Dr. Eckrich *finally* going to explore the topic of yoga, or meditation, or mindfulness, or the host of guided cognitive therapies or mood-altering medications, or aroma and phytonutrient self-help strategies for reducing the distress of anxiety and conflict and pain within our soul? As a board-certified physician, I certainly know the value of many modalities to reduce fear and anxiety, alter emotions, and assist people in coping with all sorts of distresses to their psyche or their aching physical states.

Surprise readers; I am not going into these *therapies*! If those are of further interest to you, let me refer you to my earlier book, *Fear, Anxiety and Wellness*[107], or refer you to your personal physician or mental health guide. I'm not addressing these care modalities because, frankly, they don't get at the very core reality and foundational illness harming us—the scourge of *sin* on our very body, mind, spirit—our soul—and all of creation. For this care you need God's Word, the working of God's Holy Spirit in your soul, and the ministries of those companions on your earthly journey who assist in bringing that message to you: pastors, priests, Christian educators and therapists, and your faith community.

Furthermore, in the course of any given day, you can "pause" (take a breath) and "pivot" (turn to the Spirit's leading). I invite you to incorporate these "pause and pivot" moments to help you in the care of your soul:

- Many of us within the Christian faith community make the sign of the Cross when we arise in the morning or throughout the day as a sign of our Baptismal covenant—we pause and pivot by *professing* our identity as children of God on the forehead, lips, or heart. (Romans 6:3-11)

- Daily, we pause and pivot by *placing* ourselves at the foot of the Cross, the empty Tomb, the mount of Ascension, as we enter the reading, hearing, and listening of God's Word led by the Holy Spirit to learn, mark, and inwardly digest God's loving relationship to us, and the Spirit's *processing* and *empowering* of God's will and ways to restoration through God's Son, Jesus. (2 Timothy 3:16-17; John 16:12-14)

- Daily, we are encouraged through the Scriptures to acknowledge and confess our sinfulness; ask for forgiveness and receive God's mercy—we pause and pivot by *professing* our sin, *partaking* of God's forgiveness in Word and Sacrament, and by *providing* the same forgiveness to other within our lives seeking restoration. We are called to *point* them to the Cross. (2 Corinthians 2:10; John 20:23; Matthew 18:18; 2 Corinthians 5:18; Matthew 3:6)

- Daily, we are pausing and pivoting through *prayer* focused on God's good will for us as expressed, centered, and anchored in God's Word. One form of that prayer might be meditatively praying and you can read more about that discipline in the appendix under *Word-Saturated Meditative Prayer.* (Philippians 4:6; Colossians 4:2; Acts 2:42; 1 Thessalonians 5:17; and of course, Matthew 7:7-8 and Matthew 6:5-8)

- Daily, we pause and pivot by *pondering* and *proclaiming* our faith as one's made *passively righteous* because of Christ's death. (1 Corinthians 1:30; Ephesians 1:3-14; Romans 3:21-28, 4:18-25) (See appendix under passive and active righteousness.)

- Daily, we pause and pivot by *participating actively* in that *righteousness* as we mindfully steward the gifts of our bodies, intellects, emotions, relationships, vocations, and resources. (Galatians 5:22-24; 1 Peter 4:10; Matthew 25:29; Titus 1:6-8, 2:12; Ephesians 3:1-3; Luke 16:11; Matthew 13:12, 25:23; Romans 6:19). (See the Christian Wellness Wheel on the back of this book.)

- Daily, by Christ's power, we cry defiantly in the face of Satan and all foes brought on by Sin and its sequelae displayed in an aging body, mind, and spirit—we pause and pivot by *protesting* and then *progressing* to live out our Baptismal covenant abundantly. (Romans 6:12-14; 1 John 1-2, 3:14; Galatians 3:29; 1 Corinthians 12:25)

- Daily, we pause and pivot when we acknowledge that this renewal *posture* is not of our own doing, but the *power* of Christ and his Holy Spirit, alive and working within us to mature our faith. (Titus 3:5; Philippians 3:9; Ephesians 2:8-9)

- Daily, we pause and pivot by turning from self-gain and instead *provide* thankfully and generously of our gifts and talents to God's glory and in service to God's people. (Leviticus 25:35-37; Psalm 41:1-3; Psalm 119:36; Matthew 10:42; Luke 6:37-38, 21:1-4; Acts 20:32-25)

- Keep in mind that we don't live in these disciplines because it is *necessary* for our relational wellbeing with God. We walk in these behaviors and live life together in Christ because we are joyful and thankful for God's mercy. Christ's presence, Christ's *spiritual DNA* touching, repairing, and healing our spiritual DNA, thus compels us. Participating in *discipled-lives* in and of itself does not bring resilience; these are reflections of the work God has already created in us through Christ to do. (Ephesians 2:10)

Are we within the Christian faith community living perfectly? Of course not; impossible. We know ourselves truly to be worst of sinners. (1 Timothy 1:15) But we are moved by the Spirit to walk, like the Emmaus disciples, our Baptismal journey with hearts on fire, daily. (Luke 42:33-35)

I'm a physician, so one way to consider these disciplines rather than as *resilience prescriptions* is to think of them as *wellness outcomes* of the Holy Spirit's presence, even as fruit of the Spirit's working within us. (Galatians 5:22-23) We remember our identity—who and whose we are. From our baptism and affirmation of faith on, we are *new creations* in Christ as St. Paul reminds us. (2 Corinthians 5:17)

Remembering our *wellness outcome status* is important especially when we see no other human being, or when, because of cognitive dysfunction or physical separation, we are unable to connect to others within relationships. A discipline of prayer focused in God's Word may then become the consistent conversation, connection, and link that is quintessential for our human existence.

Additionally, there may be particularly stressful circumstances that sadden and trouble our soul due to conflicted relationships within family or community. Does St. Paul provide what I might call clinical concise or "best practice" advice as to how we die to sin and rise to new life in Christ, especially in relational distress? I believe he does within his letters to the early Church.

In Ephesians 4:22-24, Paul invites us to three steps in this relational-resilience-renewal:

- "Put off your old self." This is the process of *confession,* and it involves a recognition of your deeply embedded, automated, behavioral responses to stress, fear, and challenges. (v. 22)

- "Be made new in the attitude of your minds." Through prayer, BE in Christ's presence. This requires you to do a reality check of your *self.* You need to ask is it more important to protect your personal feelings, or to be in the healing and highly valued relationship with Christ, and subsequently with the neighbor you are in conflict with. (v. 23)

- "Put on the new self, created to be like God in true righteousness and holiness." Connect the actions of the body and the thoughts of the mind to the heart of Christ, his desire to be a peaceful and non-anxious presence is our lives. Instead of being a worrywart, be "content in all things" knowing that Christ is there right in the midst of the storm. (Philippians 4:2) You then truly become the non-anxious, forgiving, and loving presence of Christ in all relationships.

And, we return to Paul for a second relational wisdom regarding resilience of our weary soul and it comes in his inspired words in Colossians 3:1-17:

> *"Therefore, as God's chosen people, holy and dearly loved, clothe yourselves with compassion, kindness, humility, gentleness and patience. Bear with each other and forgive one another if any of you has a grievance against someone. Forgive as the Lord forgave you. And over all of these virtues put on love, which binds them all together in perfect unity."*

In the end, it's all about forgiveness—forgiving as Christ has forgiven us. The act of forgiving can be so very difficult, but it is truly the beginning of healing. (Matthew 9:5) Being forgiven and sharing forgiveness softens hardened hearts, renews love, and restores a resilient soul.

Once again, we can't alter our attitude, being, or behavior by our own doing.

This is only possible through the power of the Holy Spirit building and maturing our faith, healing those damage segments of our emotional, physical, and spiritual DNA, and gradually guiding us to more Christ-like patterns of interrelating with our Creator, God's people, and all of God's creation. We are resilient because of our Redeemer! Live well in body, mind, and spirit—live well with your whole soul by his grace!

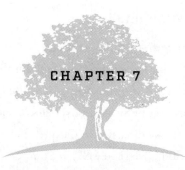

CHAPTER 7

MINDFUL WELLNESS STEWARDSHIP INTO THE NEXT SEASON OF LIFE—REPOSITIONING WITH A PURPOSE

Retirement used to be defined by working at the same career, with the same employer, in the same city, surrounded by the same friends, receiving a retirement pension, and being handed the gold watch. And then we died. That's not, generally, the same timeline today, well, except that we *will* die unless Christ comes soon and very soon.

Most Americans have a mean of 12 different job settings before they officially end their daily work career.[108] If they have been proactive in their planning and saving, and fortunate to not suffer any major disasters of health or finances—which obviously could alter their plans significantly— they should be able to "get by" until they depart this earth. In this country, we also have Social Security income to supplement our pensions and Medicare to support our health, but it is unclear how much longer these will be solvent and an assured source of fiscal foundation for those coming after us.

Quite frankly, much of what has been written about post-retirement is focused on preparing financially and subsequently wisely disbursing our resources so that they last. I think there are great guides out there and easily available through various media outlets. Please access them.

Retiring or Repositioning?

I would rather explore with you some of the other consequences, challenges, and opportunities of living longer and more functionally passed retirement *set-points*. I used that term *set-point here* as it is used in cybernetics and control theory because a set-point in those systems defines a desired or target value for the system (as we discussed in Chapter Two). The system here is life and the target is a long-lived and well-lived one, God willing. When you depart from your set-point because of a variety of variables (like disabled physical health, financial collapse, or dementia) you may not be able to fully return to stability in daily living because you can't achieve homeostasis. In other words, these disruptive forces of poor physical, cognitive, or spiritual illness may make it extremely difficult to pursue joyful and effective service in the next season of life because you have lost your *resilience*.

Even though I'm a physician, please don't consider me to be naïve or that I am implying that there are things we can *do* that will keep us alive and active *forever*. That is not in our genetic cards, and by our Christian faith, we know that the "wages of sin is death." None of us are beyond sin.

However, as I hope I have demonstrated in the previous chapters of this book, there are opportunities for us to *steward* our body, thinking, and spiritual posture, by God's grace. I believe most of us hope to maintain our resilience, our ability to be homeostatic and adaptable, beyond historically traditional *set-points* of our parents so that we can continue to love and serve God and God's creation joyfully. I believe we each have a historic opportunity to be educated, thoughtful, and mindful of how we live as we get older.

I would be remiss if I didn't address the topic of our sisters and brothers who don't get the opportunity of long life due to intervening physical or cognitive illness. There are plenty of our friends who, this very day, face a terminal illness. What incentive do they have to pursue resilience, to strive for a more responsive body, or mind, or relational capacity that could remain more able to adjust to unrelenting cancer or progressing dementia? They may well be fully cognizant of their impending death, or they may seem unaware of their lot in life, at least to our eyes.

My prayer is the same for all of us: "Lord, grant us Your comfort and mercy. We know You love us. You have promised to work all things for good. We put our trust in You. Remember us all in Your kingdom, through Christ our Savior. Let it be so."

Especially for those facing end of life decisions and terminal care, a clear recognition of the spiritual resilience gifted in Christ becomes quintessential for hope and comfort. God is faithful.

If you or your loved ones are in these circumstances, you need God's Word, the Sacraments, faith fellowship, and comfort care through pastoral ministry, hospice, or Stephen's Ministry, or many other care services available through your congregation or parish. To seek and receive this care administered under God's Word defines the very stewardship of the gifts of life. My prayer is that you pursue and connect with these ministries, and that you are simultaneously surrounded by a cloud of saints from your faith community lifting you to God's throne of grace and mercy.

On the other hand, if God grants you the opportunity to live beyond your expected career limits, what are the questions we might ask yourself and other loved ones around you to help you repurpose and energize for this next season of life?

Before exploring these curious and vital questions, let me make one further and most emphatic point about aging. This point was brought home to me with a steady eye and a thoughtful mind of an elderly patient of mine I visited several years ago in a nursing home. This beautiful lady was well into her 80s and now hobbled by rheumatoid arthritis which limited the most simple of daily tasks and basically confined her to her bed.

"Anna," I said, "God has continued to bless you with a wonderfully active and clear mind, even though I know it is tough for you to get around much these days. I hear from so many of your students about how much of an impact you made in their lives. Don't you miss your career as a teacher?" Obviously, I must have tweaked an especially lively set of nerve synapses in that highly functional mind. With a bright twinkle and unwavering voice, Anna replied, "Doc, I can't do much these days...but I can talk to God; I can still pray!" Indeed, Anna understood the vitality and power of prayer.

"I can still remember my class list for each first grade I taught, and I just spend my time talking to God about each one of those children." Pretty much at a loss for words at this point, I asked her, "Well, what do you ask God to do for them?" "Give them joy wherever and whatever they are doing, of course!" she responded. Of course.

The good Lord has a plan and a purpose for each of us, beyond retirement, and up to the point of our death—that is my firm belief as a person of faith. As I frequently recall, "we know that in all things God works for the good of those who love him, who have been called according to his purpose." (Romans 8:28) Short life, long life; vigorously active or limited to a wheelchair or an extended care facility; sharp cognition, or fuzzy; I believe God has and invites us to a vision and a purpose for our lives.

But if you have been granted with some additional time, how do you go about figuring out what to do with it? Frankly, there are substantial resources on aging strategies just as there are grand financial guidebooks for growing old. Again, I invite you to explore good book stores or websites or pick your colleagues' brains for specific help. What about insuring your healthcare dollar? Here is one more simple addition to your "maturing" portfolio to consider.

Healthcare Planning in Repositioning

There is one aspect of wellness and aging that I find critical to address for all of us— health insurance. The price tag for healthcare in the United States is staggering and I have observed and experienced that as both a provider and consumer. Many of us have had that coverage as a benefit of employment, so in a sense we may not fully comprehend the actual cost; others have had to purchase healthcare coverage out of pocket in after tax dollars periodically or all along our working years. If you're in that later category, you may already understand the financial burden you may be facing after retirement or the retirement of your spouse if that is the source of your coverage. It can easily consume 15-30% of your yearly income for adequate insurance.

Therefore, in addition to taking into account our 401(k)s, pension plans, social security checks, and savings plans, etc., a significant assessment of healthcare insurance (long and short term) is time well spent. If you are fortunate, your employer will have a well-versed and easily accessed advisory service to help you in your transition to Medicare, Medicaid, and Medicare-supplement offerings. You, however, are you own best healthcare advocate, so you need to be proactive and aggressive in understanding and establishing a good continuum of healthcare coverage.

Additionally, there are private insurance brokers who can guide you through your coverage decisions, but at a cost.

Here are just a few suggestions:

- Begin the insurance transition early, if possible *a year* before your planned retirement. Ask questions, gather options, read everything your employer sends you regarding retirement, and reread everything a second time.

- Visit your Social Security/Medicare office again at least 3-4 months prior to retirement to understand the details of transitioning to Medicare, the personal out-of-pocket costs you might face, and the costs to your spouse if they are also to receive Medicare and

Social Security. Additionally, if your yearly income exceeds certain income thresholds (only about 5% of beneficiaries) you may also face additional Medicare costs called Income Related Monthly Adjustment Amounts (IRMAA) on both Part B doctor coverage and Part D drug coverage.

- Make sure to correlate the *date* that your employer healthcare coverage ceases and Medicare begins, especially noting to the Medicare office the date that Medicare becomes your *primary health insurance* and your Medicare supplement becomes *secondary*.

- Make sure you have health cards for all insurances and that your physicians' offices, clinics, or hospitals have all of the proper health insurance coverage well and accurately documented.

- Keep regularly scheduled appointments with your physicians; preventive care matters.

- Consider procuring long-term care insurance as early in life as you are able. Let alone physician, medication, and hospitalization costs which can overwhelm us, the need for assisted living or skilled nursing home care can devastate even the best laid plans for retirement for you, your spouse, or both of you. You can completely erase any hope for financial legacy for your loved ones with just a year or two in extended care facilities. Even though it seems like "another insurance bill" at a time when income is fixed in retirement, long-term care insurance can be relatively affordable and comparatively a bargain compared to assuming the full cost of aging care in well-staffed facilities. Have that conversation with your trustworthy insurance adviser and your family.

A Written Planner for the Next Season

Now that you have read this book and have a baseline understanding of what changes in body, mind, and spirit with age and have a few solid suggestions on how to preserve and enhance function, I would urge you to begin this search with a series of practical questions. Why not grab a pen or pencil and fill in some of the blanks for reference points:

What gives you joy? _____

_____

_____

What brings you energy or resilience; what renews you? _____

_____

_____

What speaks to your passions? _____

_____

_____

Given limited time or resources, what appears to you to be worth the effort? _____

_____

_____

What could be a legacy to give to your family? _____

_____

_____

What do you perceive God is calling you to do with your gifts, talents, and passions? _____

_____

What are you equipped adequately to accomplish? Do you need more education, training, resources? _____

_____

What would be something needed by your family or community that you have the unique ability to accomplish? _____

_____

What will you have to sacrifice to make your new purpose a reality?

_____

_____

Are you happier being a leader or a follower? Do you want to work outside or inside? Are you physically functional enough to accomplish your vision? What do other people profess that you do very well?

_____

_____

Are you dealing with specific physical or cognitive challenges? If so, listing them may help clarify areas to explore for developing resilience; document below: _____

_____

Here are a few projects that might require others to provide you with a helping hand:

Consult pastor, social workers, or educational resources that have experience in gerontology. Attend seminars given by reputable resources (not just someone trying to sell you a financial package). What seminars or resources are being offered near you or via Internet? _____

_____

_____

Incorporate spiritual and altruistic concepts into your plan. List a few of these that come to mind: _____ .

_____

_____

Consult and keep your family and close friends involved in your decisions and activities to serve both as sustainers but also resources to help you keep to your goals. List some significant members of your support team: _____

_____

_____

_____

Have accessory purposes to your hobbies. If you love golf, try to find opportunities to walk, not just ride in the cart. Choose brain-strengthening exercises like cards, memory-based, or problem-solving strategies. Write down a few examples that come to mind: _____

_____

Get a good doctor and do it before you turn 65. Many physicians are not accepting new Medicare patients. List your healthcare providers:

_____

_____

You can find a list of all my current medications at: _____

_____

Do you have a financial advisory team and attorneys? If so, please list:

_____

_____

_____

My will and/or living trust is written, certified or notarized, and can be found securely kept at: _____

_____

I have a durable power of attorney for financial matters, and it can be found at: _____

_____

I have a durable power of attorney for healthcare and it can be found at: _____

_____

I have written instructions regarding my wishes for artificially supplied respiration, hydration, and nutrition (often included in a durable power of attorney for healthcare), which can be found at:

_____

_____

I have my health insurance coverage for the next season in life in place.

My primary health coverage is: _____

_____

Secondary (Supplemental) coverage is: _____

ID #: _____

I have long-term care insurance through: _____

_____

I have preplanned funeral arrangements and they can be found at:

_____

_____

_____

I hope these questions provide a guide of worthwhile data points to form the basis of conversations with family, friends, and the good Lord regarding the "what's next" planning that should follow the reading of this text. I believe those are valuable discussions to help you make wise decisions and satisfying choices.

As one aging with you, let me offer you this blessing. Age with peace. Age with joy. Age gracefully. Age with renewed purpose. Mindfully steward your whole being. Serve and care for God's people and God's whole creation. Fear, love, and trust the Lord with your whole being, with your soul.

APPENDIX

HISTORICAL PERSPECTIVES ON BEING HUMAN

THE BLUE ZONE SPECIFICS

INCURVATUS IN SE

CHALLENGING QUESTIONS ABOUT THE SOUL

WHEN DOES THE SOUL BEGIN?

WHY IS THE SOUL CREATED?

DOES THE SOUL SLEEP IN DEATH?

WHAT HAPPENS TO THE SOUL AT DEATH? A DISCUSSION OF PURGATORY AND GRACE

WHAT DOES CHRISTIAN THEOLOGY TEACH REGARDING DUALISM? UNDERSTANDING A SEPARATE BODY AND MIND/SOUL VS. MONISM (INSEPARABLE BODY AND MIND/SOUL)

WHAT DOES JESUS TELL US ABOUT THE SOUL? THE CONTEXT OF JESUS' MINISTRY, AGING AND HIS END OF LIFE TEACHINGS

HOW DOES THE SOUL FIT INTO THE DOCTRINE OF LAW AND GOSPEL?

DOES THE SOUL AGE? THE THEOLOGY OF PASSIVE AND ACTIVE RIGHTEOUSNESS

IS THE SOUL UNIQUELY HUMAN?

WORD-SATURATED MEDITATIVE PRAYER

HISTORICAL PERSPECTIVES ON BEING HUMAN

For many decades, at least within medical, sociological, and theological circles, we have tried to explain the characteristics of humankind by teaching that the human being is made of distinct components rather than a mysterious, unified whole. We are said to be made of either two (body-soul) or three elements (a body, a mind, and a soul or spirit). I alluded to this in primary text. And we often interchange the words *spirit* and *soul*.

Is this *compartmentalization* of humanness into components because we are really a complex, two- or three-part creature in which two or three elements co-exist, are integrated, and interact with each other to make up the *whole* person? Or are we trying to compartmentalize our human natures so that we can better understand, evaluate, and treat function and dysfunction in an effort to assert some control over our whole mysterious selves? I suspect some combination of both strategies along with some you yourself might add for understanding humanity is helpful and valuable.

This *division* verses *unification* of the component content of humanness has recurrently permeated and promulgated discourse throughout the ages. It may be instructive to explore historically a few thoughts on what it means to be human. By using both archeological and textual resources over the last 5,000 years we can gain perspective on being human from some of the more ancient philosophies in the early cultures of India, China, and Egypt. Their viewpoints appear to trickle into much of the *humanism* we talk of today.

Humanness in Hinduism

Hinduism defines being human in a functional sense by saying that humanness is "service to mankind and that is the same as service to God." Body, mind, and spirit are integrally tied to being in service to others as a whole being. Being human is primarily a relational concept, how we relate to God and to fellow creations of God. A *devotional servanthood posture* is what cultivates goodness and humility, making us human, and is what differentiates us from the rest of creation. Servanthood also moves us to reach a supreme dwelling place with God—being at the same level as God.[109]

Humanness in Confucianism

Confucians (Confucius living 551-479 BCE) use the word *ren* to define humanness, mature love, or altruism. Confucians historically view each person "not as a morally autonomous individual but as a social being whose identity derives from his interaction with and conduct within the broader human community." To display *ren* (humanness) requires aging with maturity. Here again we see humanness based in relationships and relational goodness. Later Confucian writers like Mencius (371-289 BCE) teach that *ren* comes from feeling compassion and commiseration within both the human heart and mind so that there are both affective and cognitive components involved. When those mind and heart feelings lead to physical action, then *ren* is brought to wholeness or fruition.[110]

Several subsequent Chinese philosophies, including *Daoism,* lessen the status of humanness, introducing a concept that humans are only one class of things among many in creation, rather than placing humanness above other aspects of creation.[111]

Humanness for Ancient Egyptians

Ancient Egyptians believed that the human is a soul made up of five parts: the *Ren,* the *Ba,* the *Ka,* the *Sheut,* and the *Jb.* These components uniquely carry emotion, thought, and will into the afterlife.[112] Even a person's name extends life after death as long as the name is spoken. Vital essence (animation) is breathed into the human by a variety of gods at birth but require food and drink in the afterlife to sustain them.[113]

A final component of human life and death in Egyptian thought is the *Akh. Akh* is associated with thought, but not an action of the mind; rather, it is intellect as a living entity. After death, the *Ba* and the *Ka* are reunited to reanimate the *Akh*. It is the concept of a ghost or roaming dead being. The *Akh* can cause nightmares, feelings of guilt, and even form sicknesses, and can be influenced by prayers or appeals to inflict punishments of have positive influence on situations and other living beings.[114]

Humanness in Western Thought

Prior to the Athenian Socrates (d. 399 BCE), the Greek philosopher Protagoras wrote that being human meant "being the reference point from which all else is known." Therefore we had to use a variety of definitions to describe what it meant to be human. Scientifically, the Greeks said that a human being was a complex biological organism belonging in the great ape family labeled *Homo sapiens*. It meant we were self-aware, used language and learning, abstract thought, and logical reasoning. We could solve complex problems, create advanced technology, and develop and exist in complex social institutions.

Whether in modern English, old German, Norse, or Franconian, the root word for the *soul* seems to come from the concept of *coming from or belonging to the sea or lake*. Greek ascribes a *cooling or blowing from the breath* to the definition of soul giving the soul characteristics of a spirit, life, or consciousness.

Ancient Greek philosophers used the term *alive* to signify being a person who is *ensouled*. For the Greeks, the *soul* is the *spiritual breath* that enlivens the body. But the Greeks described that *ensouled-state* as being only perceived through the body's *animation*.

The School of Athens colleagues, Plato and Aristotle, envisioned the soul as the *essence* of a person that defines how a being *behaves*. Their predecessor, Socrates, taught that the soul lives on even after death and is able to continue to think, and is continually reborn in other bodies.

Plato refined the thoughts about the composition of the soul into three distinct components:

- Logos: mind or reason—resides in the head Thymos: emotion or the masculine—resides near the chest and is related to anger

- Eros: desire or the feminine—resides in the stomach as is related to one's desires

Each part of the soul interacts with the others so that the human being functions in harmony. However, the *logos* is the *regulator* of the other two parts of the soul.[115]

Aristotle, living 300 years BCE, defined the soul as inseparable from the body; form and function are one in the same. The soul is the *organization* of the being that allows it to function fully as a human. Further, Aristotle defined a hierarchy of three levels to living beings (all of which he believed have souls): *plants*, which possess *vegetative souls* purposed for reproduction and growth; *animals*, which possess *sensitive souls* for sensation and movement; and *humans*, who possess *rational souls* made for thought and reflection.

Students of early Greek philosophers wrestle with whether Aristotle professed a mortal or immortal soul in humans. In his writings, it is reasonable to believe that he considers the soul as a whole to be mortal, but a portion of the soul, which might be called *the active intellect or mind,* to be considered eternal and immortal. These arguments are found in his work *De Anima* or *On the Soul.*[116]

Some early philosophers even suggest that the soul sleeps while the body is awake, but that the soul awakens within our dreams.[117] We will touch on *soul-sleep* later in the appendix.

THE BLUE ZONE SPECIFICS

For those who want to have more information on the health habits of people who live within the five Blue Zones, a summary of key points from the various Blue Zone books in included here.[10, 11]

Ikaria, Greece

This beautiful island sits in the Aegean Sea. It houses one of the world's lowest rates of middle-age mortality and the lowest rates of dementia. This may be, in large part, related to the Ikarian diet.

There is great interest in many health circles over the advantages of *The Mediterranean Diet*. Food choices in Ikaria kitchens are a microcosm of this style of eating. The Ikarian diet is rich in vegetables, especially greens, beans, and fruit. Their diet has about 50% of their calories as fat, but more than half of that fat comes from the use of extra virgin olive oil with its fine unsaturated vegetable fat content. About 5% of their diet comes from meat, and 6% from fish, with its great omega-3 fatty acids. They consume colored vegetables like arugula with its wonderful content of carotenoids. Ikarians do consume potatoes almost daily, which helps reduce blood pressure, diabetes, and is a wonderful anti-inflammatory.

You don't find a lot of electric mixers and mashers in an Ikarian kitchen. Most of the cooking is done by hand rather than with the help of modern appliances. Bread is kneaded by muscle power, allowed to rise over night with the same bacteria that had fermented great-great-grandmothers' fine sourdough; traditional food, traditional ingredients, traditional preparation.

Typical ingredients include goat's milk (and the anti-inflammatory and gut-friendly feta cheese), potatoes, beans (garbanzos, black-eyed peas, and lentils), honey for sweetening, greens, a little fruit, and a little fish. The lack of cow's milk, and preference for goat dairy, has been shown in several studies to reduce coronary artery disease. Olive oil probably lowers bad cholesterol (LDL) and increases good cholesterol (HDL). The wild greens have ten times more antioxidants than wine, and yet red wine in moderation helps the body absorb more of the flavonoids, which are the artery-scrubbing antioxidants in the food we eat. Plus, Ikarians put lemon juice on everything, helping to benefit blood sugar and diabetes.

The Ikarians like their coffee, and like it strong—Turkish-style. We are seeing more and more studies suggesting lower rates of diabetes, heart disease, and even reduced rates of Parkinson's disease in coffee drinkers. Ikarians also prefer tea brewed from wild mint (prevents gingivitis), rosemary to treat gout, and Artemisia (daisy family) to spark blood circulation. These herbs are filled with antioxidants as well as prove to be wonderful diuretics; this lowers BP and removes body wastes.

Perhaps equally important to the specific foods consumed on Ikaria is the fact that Ikarians eat food from their own gardens, *sans* the chemicals of industrially grown produce.

Their natural greens and even some products we might consider weeds in the US, like dandelion, chicory, and wild fennel, are filled with vitamins A, C, and K; potassium and iron, magnesium and calcium; and they are loaded with fiber.

Meat is an infrequent component of meals. Ikarians eat meat only once or twice a week. They may share a small amount of poultry weekly, but more often may use salted cod or sardines, and more rarely fresh caught fish. They eat little dessert.

There are a few other notable health habits of Ikarians. They eat slowly and with family or friends, rarely alone. They nap frequently, and 80% of Ikarian males between 65 and 85 were still having sex.

Sardinia, Italy

If you visit any nursing home in the U.S., you will find inhabitants are predominantly women. *"Where have all the young men gone?"* to paraphrase a Sixties hit by Peter, Paul, and Mary.

Sardinia distinguishes itself by having and inordinate number of men living past 100, a far greater percentage than anywhere else in the world. In the US, only one in 5,000 males live to 100. In the mountainous Ogliastra region of Sardinia, five centenarians are living among the 2,500 inhabitants.

Many of these men shepherd the sheep and goats that dot the hillsides. This is rugged work with hearty men tending, protecting, carrying, milking, and butchering the flock for sustenance. A fourth of their diet comes from dairy (pecorino cheese with high omega-3's), and half of the intake is made up of grains, with lots of barley and its much lower glycemic index. The shepherds also consume a modest amount of wine daily. Their food is laced with fennel, a licorice-flavored vegetable with high levels of vitamins A, B, and C. Fava beans and chickpeas deliver lots of protein and fiber. Rich tomatoes, with potassium and vitamin C, top many pizzas and breads.

Incidentally, their sheep and goats appear to be rather skinny lot in that they only consumed grass and herbs. Therefore the animals are hardly worth butchering but are mostly used to provide the dairy so predominant in Sardinian diets.

The ratio of men to women over 100 is one-to-one. Women aren't dying sooner; men are just living longer by fighting off heart disease. Most likely, men face less day-to-day stress in that the women are the home-keepers, child-rearers, and chief financial officers of the family funds, meager as they are. As one Sardinian woman said of her husband, "He works. I worry."

Furthermore, no one *retires* in Sardinia. They repurpose; they contribute to society through continuing to be active and continuing to engage their brains in the health of the family and community. Families live multi-generationally; they care for the aged at home. To do otherwise would bring shame to the family.

The shepherd activity of hill-climbing appears to be key to long life. This provides low-intensity, slow, and regular muscle activity. There are no treadmills and Gold's Gyms in the villages of Sardinia.

Finally, the researchers studying Sardinian diet discover that more than 65% of daily calories come from carbohydrates like pastas, flat breads (barley more than wheat), potatoes, and beans. Fat intake comes mostly from goat's milk or sheep's cheese, but also from olive oil. Most of their protein came from beans. Meat, often pigs or chickens, are holiday treats. Because Sardinians live in the high mountains far from the sea, even though they are on an island, they rarely consume fish. They take three to four small glasses of wine per day. Their wine is a distinctive garnet-red color made from Grenache grapes, stressed by the hot sun.

Tragically, as transportation and electricity have begun to flow more readily into Sardinia since WWII, the younger generation has added more frozen foods, more meat, and probably diminished the intensity of daily physical labor. Researchers are finding increased rates of obesity, diabetes, and heart disease in the population born since the 1940s.

Okinawa, Japan

On the island cluster south of Japan lies an ancient culture filled with long-lived people, descendants of the Ryukyu kingdom. In fact, if you are an Okinawan over the age 65, you have the longest life expectancy on earth. Men live into their mid-80s and women to 90+; in fact, the world's longest-living women are Okinawans. More importantly, they suffer half the rate of dementia as Americans, a fifth of the heart disease, and a fifth the rate of our prostate and breast cancer. That's impressive.

What might account for the healthy longevity? The first clue might be the heavy dependency of those living before the 1940s on the *imo,* a purple or yellow variety of the sweet potato (high in vitamin C, flavonoids, fiber, carotenoids, and with a low glycemic index). This tuber was brought to the islands from the Americas nearly 400 years ago, and thankfully it thrived, otherwise the Okinawans might have starved to death before WWII.

Also before the Second World War, the Okinawans ate fish three times per week, large quantities of vegetables (80% imo-based), and simple grains. They also ate soy filled with flavonoids in the form of tofu. They rarely ate meat, except in special festival days, and then usually the family pig. Of note is that the pork consumed had been cooked for days and the fat recurrently skimmed off. They were really eating high-protein collagen. Incidentally, pork protein is very similar to human protein. Actually, it may have been acting like a little caulking compound to patch tears in small arteries like in the brain.

They enjoyed miso soup (seaweed) which also contained their imo and tofu. Their main dish of the day was predominantly vegetable-based containing a bitter melon called goya (good antidiabetic), radishes, okra, pumpkin, root vegetables, and perhaps a small amount of meat or fish. They drank predominantly a jasmine tea. Furthermore, they also consumed turmeric with extraordinary anti-inflammatory benefits we are discovering today. All in all, they were probably consuming 40% fewer calories than a typical American diet.

Frankly, they were often in a starvation mode, and this calorie-restricted diet provided the benefits of having their cells self-protect by throwing off fewer free radicals (radicals causing premature aging in the skin, arteries, and brain). The fact that their diet included substantial amounts of sweet potatoes, seaweed, and turmeric, however, provided within themselves a reduction of free radicals—a double bang for the caloric-buck!

However, here's the troubling news for modern Okinawans, and we can thank the influence of our country for much of the new Okinawan dietary culture. During and after WWII, with much influence from the American bases established on these islands, traditional food habits changed. Sweet potato consumption has dropped from 60% to less than 5% of calories. Bread, rice, and milk consumption is rising sharply. Eggs, meat, and poultry products are increasing sevenfold. Colon, breast, and lung cancer also are rising dramatically.

Even though fast-food restaurants now abound in Okinawa, a most fascinating residual of the American forces occupying Okinawa is the predominance of Spam (brought in the U.S. rations) still prevalent today. Cultures, particularly in their diets, change slowly.

Fortunately, Okinawans still eat plenty of tofu (soy), which lowers cholesterol and triglycerides; garlic (helping prevent aging), turmeric (as spice in foods and as tea with dramatic anti-inflammatory properties); jasmine tea with turmeric; shitake mushrooms (more than 100 immune-protective properties); and brown rice (superb ability to breakdown carbohydrates and proteins).

Nicoya Peninsula, Costa Rica

In the hilly region of Costa Rica lies a rather isolated strip of land called the Nicoya Peninsula. The people living there are a complex mixture of native Chorotega Indians, Spanish colonists, and African slaves. The 21st century has come slowly to Nicoya, in most recent decades influenced by the contras, US-backed counterrevolutionaries mounting resistance to the Nicaraguan Sandinistas. Nicoya has the world's lowest rates of middle-age mortality, and the second-highest concentration of male centenarians.

Tropical infections previously were dominating the death scrolls including dysentery, diarrhea, malaria, and dengue fever. Despite the ominous bugs, middle-aged men here are living past 90 far more often than in the US. There is much less cancer, heart disease, and diabetes, and this is in the shadow of far less healthcare.

The National Geographic team discovered that the power and strength of their faith community, the constant low-level physical exertion, and their deep social networks are major contributors to the people's wellbeing. Even with the amount of dengue fever which is known to produce "broken bone disease," they obtain high doses of calcium in their water supply and spend copious amounts of time in the sun to obtain vitamin D. Perhaps there are fewer fatal falls in the aged.

The Nicoyan diet also has more carbohydrates than the American diet, up to 68%. Most of their carbs come from beans (again), rice, and maize. The diets are relatively low in protein, and fat is about 20% of intake. They consume around 1,800 calories per day, compared to American consumption nearing 2,700 calories per day.

As in the other Blue Zones, the diet here is low-calorie, low-fat, plant-focused, and filled with beans. They also eat lots of tropical fruits like sweet oranges and lemons, bananas, and daily maize tortillas, hand-made, and filled with niacin. They also love a variety of squash most like pumpkins, butternut, and spaghetti squash filled with carotenoids. Their daily diet is an extraordinary cardiac cocktail raising HDL (good cholesterol) and lowering LDL (bad cholesterol). Their agricultural crop planting tradition allows for soil conservation and preservation of nitrogen in the soil.

Papayas, which grow naturally in the Costa Rican hillsides, are consumed daily. These fruits are filled with vitamins A, C, and E and are loaded with papain, a powerful anti-inflammatory. Likewise a true Costa Rican yam loaded with B6 is a staple. Furthermore, black beans concentrated with antioxidants are combined with rice, squash, and corn tortillas.

A multitude of bananas and plantains rich in carbs, potassium, and soluble fiber are consumed as part of everyday meals or as snacks. Peach palms filled with vitamins A and C are boiled then served chilled.

Loma Linda, California

The only American Blue Zone can be found in the foothills ascending to the snowcapped San Jacinto Mountains of Southern California. Loma Linda is a relatively younger city being incorporated only in 1970 with a population of around 25,000. Its roots, however, extend back to a health resort called Mound City.

Loma Linda is the home to one of the largest concentrations of Seventh Day Adventists in the world. This religious denomination is distinguished by adhering to a very strict Biblical diet characterized by *vegetarianism.* They also place a ban on smoking city-wide and have strict rules governing the sale of alcohol. The church-owned grocery store does not sell meat.

The healthcare of Loma Linda is anchored in the Loma Linda University Medical Center. It is an outstanding Level One trauma center and has a wide variety of medical training programs including medicine, dentistry, nursing, pharmacy, and behavioral and public health. You might recall the pioneering pediatric heart transplant story of Baby Fae, who as an infant who received a heart transplanted from a baboon in 1984 by Dr. Leonard Bailey. Though Baby Fae died shortly thereafter, this procedure led to successful programs of pediatric heart surgery around the world.

Of interest to the Blue Zone researchers and of interest to us is the fact that Seventh Day Adventists tend to live longer than any other Americans. The Adventists are a very conservative Protestant group who evangelize with health activities and celebrate the Sabbath on Saturday in the traditional Jewish manner, rather than Sunday.

Sunset Friday until sunset Saturday is "sanctuary time." The Adventists spend nearly 24 hours in attending church, being with family, and spend much time in quiet contemplation. They use this precious weekly time to avoid TV, movies, or other distractions. After Saturday church they join other Adventists in potluck lunches, followed by nature walks, sunshine, and fresh air. Generally, they avoid drinking, smoking, and dancing.

Their diet is taken straight out of the Old Testament as they cite Genesis 1:29: "And God said, behold, I have given you every herb bearing seed, which is upon the face of all the earth, and every tree, in the which is the fruit of a tree yielding see; to you it shall be for meat." In fact, most Christian theologians suggest that the consumption of animal meat for common food does not occur until after the Flood. (Genesis 6-9)

Adventists consume a well-balanced diet with 27% fruits; 33% vegetables; legumes and soy 12%; nuts and seeds 2%; grains 7%; dairy about 10%; meat and poultry 4%, and fish and eggs 1% each. They do prohibit "unclean" meat like pork and shellfish. The only liquid consumed is water, and they encourage at least 6 glasses per day. If you review this diet, you will also note it is very low in salt, sugar, and refined grains. There is little consumption of coffee and minimal alcohol. Therefore there is very little obesity, and extremely low rates of heart disease and diabetes.

Adventists live up to a decade longer than the rest of us Americans. Here is a list of the probable key factors from studies of Adventists funded by the National Institutes of Health:

- A plant-slant diet with small amounts of dairy and fish
- No smoking
- Maintenance of medium body weight
- Eating a handful of nuts four to five times per week
- Regular physical activity

Furthermore recent studies of the Seventh Day Adventists reported in the National Geographic's Special Blue Zone Publication found that people who eat more meat also tend to ingest more soft drinks, desserts, and refined grains, and as a result, tend to be heavier. However, rigid vegetarians were not the ones living the longest; that distinction went to pesco-vegetarians—those who eat a plant-based diet with up to one serving of fish per day. Hooray for omega-3 fatty acids!

INCURVATUS IN SE

The Christian faith teaches that in our natural state we are turned away from our relationship with our Creator and turned into ourselves. *Incurvatus in se* is the Latin phrase traditionally used within Christianity to define sin. It simply means that humans prefer to place *Me (myself above all)* before *We (God and my relationship with God above all).* But what does this inwardness have to do with resilient aging or aging in general?

Being inward-focused and self-centered has been the fundamental motion and orientation of humankind since the entrance of sin into God's creation. Evolutionists might suggest that this inward direction is essential for *the survival of the fittest.* Christians on-the-other-hand understand that this tendency is at the very core of the separation of creation from its Creator and therefore marks the beginning of life's eventual spiral within the *wages of sin* which ends in death.

This self-destruction permeates body, mind, and spirit. Consider these examples:

Body: By placing *Me* before *We,* we tend to:

- focus our body-care behavior on satisfying personal needs and desires by drinking alcohol or eating sugar-laden, fatty foods that exceed basic caloric needs

- avoid movement and exercise because it's "hard," raises a sweat, and takes too much time away from *my pleasure*

- place personal ease over concern for society by wastefully expending our earth's bounty for the good of ourselves rather than the good of all

By not being good stewards of these wellness gifts from God to creation, we see the deleterious results in bodies less able to withstand the natural changes and stress that accompany age, including narrow blood vessels, poor immunity, arthritis, cancer, and diabetes.

Mind: By placing Me before We, we tend to:

- engage in addictive behavior, emotions, and feelings aimed at pleasing ourselves at the expense of our family or society

- ruminate and become anxious over how a relationship or circumstance satisfies our desires rather than considering the needs and feelings of those close to us

- close or constrict our communication with loved ones because with age we don't hear, see, or speak with the same acuity we did when we were younger and often isolate ourselves from meaningful interactions because we fear being less valued and less worthy because of our disabilities

Consider this illustration of an aging left side of the brain and a younger right side. The left aging brain is compartmentalized, each activity confined to its own cubicle without effective intra-compartmental communication. In contrast, the right young brain shows the free, enjoyable, effective, and active flow of ideas and memories that define the function of a healthy brain. It is also a picture of how an aging, dementia-prone brain with its tangles and bundles of poorly integrated wiring functions compares to a brain with healthy cognition.

Spirit: By placing *Me* before *We,* we tend to:

- place ourselves as equal or above our Creator, as seen in numerous Scriptural examples: Adam and Eve (Genesis 3); Cain and Abel (Genesis 4); Joseph and his brothers (Genesis 37); King David and Bathsheba (2 Samuel 11); Jesus and his disciples (Mark 10:35-45); the early Church (2 Corinthians 8-9).

- fear, love, or trust ourselves above God and thereby separate ourselves from being God's sons and daughters; we reject God's grip

Aging Brain vs. Young Brain

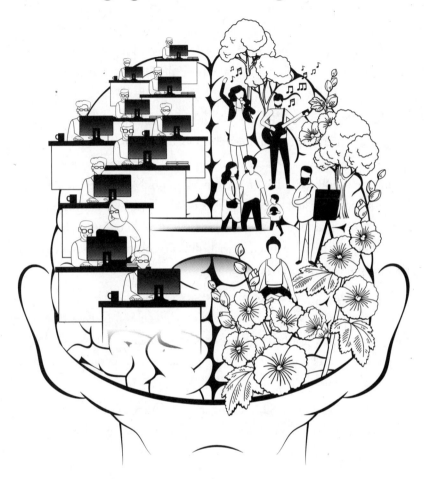

of grace in our lives, refuse what God's Son has done for us on the Cross, and close ourselves to the working of the Holy Spirit in our hearts

When turned inward on ourselves, our physical behaviors, thoughts and emotions, and spiritual tenets will harm and constrict the vitality, effectiveness, longevity, and joy of our lives. St. Paul gives us in Romans 7:15, 18-19 a perfect description of incurvatus in se:

"For that which I do I allow not: for what I would, that do I not; but what I hate, that I do. For I know that in me (that is, in my flesh,) dwelleth no good thing: for to will is present with me; but how to perform that which is good I find not. For the good that I would I do not: but the evil which I would not, that I do." (KJV)

Both St. Augustine of Hippo (who may have coined the term *incurvatus in se*) and particularly Martin Luther expound in depth on this idea in their writings. (See Luther's *Lectures on Romans*.) Luther describes this *first sin* as "being too deeply curved in on itself that it not only bends the best gifts of God towards itself and enjoys them (as is plain in the *works-righteous* and hypocrites), or rather even uses God himself in order to attain these gifts, but it also fails to realize that it so wickedly, curvedly, and viciously seeks all things, even God, for its own sake."[118]

Theologian Karl Barth later extends a description of sin that goes beyond the sin of pride. He writes of *simul justus et peccator* and explains that even though people are justified by Jesus' death on the Cross, they still have the propensity to sin against God because they are simultaneously both *saint* (justified) and *sinner*.[119]

The meaning is clear. Sin, turning inward, touches every corner of the human experience and is the root cause of our aging and our demise.

WHEN DOES THE SOUL *BEGIN?*

We have no indication from the Scriptures that the Creator has a warehouse of *souls or spirits* from which God picks one and inserts it into a material body. Just as Adam and Eve were created as whole beings, we too are created—body, mind, and spirit—a complete soul at the point of conception—as whole beings.

We have evidence that some biochemical, inter-atomic interactions might be able to explain some of the *psychological* or *emotional* components of human behavior just as they do physical activity. However, there remains a mysterious nature of humankind beyond the material matter. There is that which *binds* or *coheres* the whole together, the *religio* (Latin). What might that *religio* or that *binder* be? I believe the Scriptures speak to that in the First Commandment: *fear, love, and trust of God and God's promise.* Our whole being must ultimately fear, love, and trust a relational Creator and Sustainer God. That posture allows us to dare or prevents us from daring to make choices; to do things or not do them; to live consistent with or in opposition to God's good will for us as God's creation.

Ethically, medically, and culturally, there are those who would argue that *wholeness* or having *living-being-status* only occurs at the point that an embryo can be potentially living outside the womb; at least in this country, medical and political opinion places that at the beginning of the third trimester when there appears to be a reasonable chance that a child can survive even if on a respirator and with massive perinatal support. Incidentally, *whose* womb, or test tube, or petri dish, or incubator, or freezer, I would ask? Further, there are others who would posit that a *living being* only comes at the point of *delivery* from the womb, at birth, by vaginal or caesarian delivery. Traditional orthodox Christian stance places that origin at fertilization of egg with sperm.

Dramatically, we see these timing-definitions being used to support or denounce *life-choice decisions*. However, science is continuously pushing the envelope at all points along the womb-viability-birth-life-death time spectrum. Relying on *viability at birth* as the definition of *living being*, or of the timing of *spirit joining the body*, remains highly troublesome at so many scientific, medical, and theological levels. There are myriad volumes of research and public discourse which propose to support or undercut whatever argument you might wish to use for making life prolonging or terminating decisions regarding your own life or the lives of others. I'll share with you my view as a physician, scientist, and Christian: the point of creation of a whole being as being conception—or the joining of egg and sperm—remains the surest marker for defining a quintessential event for *human life*, despite the moral quagmire that such a definition might present to some in our culture. In an earth bound by time, it is the surest indicator for the human life of *zero hour*, the *moment of truth*.

Is that the instant that a boundless, non-time-constrained Creator breathes into the dust of a mortal being God's breath or spirit? I don't know; that's the best answer I can offer.

I think I can safely say, however, that a human being cannot be a *whole being* without this initial, God-ordained step of the joining of a mother's egg and the father's seed. The rest of the human story, we get to ask God face to face at the Judgment.

WHY IS THE SOUL CREATED?

The human creature is made with cause and design: stewardship—multiple, fill the earth, care for it, subdue it...and be vegetarian! (Genesis 1:29) God doesn't let us be "meatetarians" until after the Flood. (Genesis 9:3) Adam and Eve are made in the *image and likeness of God*, instilled with the capacity to *fear, love and trust* their Creator, and that includes the capacity to follow and steward God's rules and order for creation. (Genesis 2-3) Eve appears to be made after Adam but of the same basic DNA and purpose. (Genesis 2:20-23) Additionally, she is to become the mother of all the living humans. (Genesis 3:20)

As stated above, our Creator has purpose, knowledge, and vision for our whole being as God works from eternity, but down into a time-framed creation. "For we are God's workmanship, created in Christ Jesus to do good works, which God prepared in advance for us to do." (Ephesians 2:10)

Let's flesh out this purpose for humankind a bit more. What might be the reason(s) for creating a *whole being*; what do we know of *purpose* directly from God's mouth to us in the Scriptures?

- You are created to *know* God—to be in *relationship* with God, and that comes through our relationship with God's Son, Jesus. (John 3:3; John 6:35; John 14:6; Romans 10:9-10)

- You are created to *glorify* God—to praise and worship God. (Psalm 86:9; 12)

- You are created to *grow in the fruit of the Spirit*—maturing in love, joy, peace, patience, kindness, goodness, faithfulness, gentleness, and self-control. (Galatians 5:22-23)

- You are created to *tell others the good news of restoration and salvation in Christ*. (Isaiah 12:4; Matthew 28:19-20)

- You are created to *steward and use the gifts* God gave you. (Romans 12:4-8)

- You are created to be God's child. (Galatians 3:26)

Despite our continuous propensity as humans to screw up God's purpose and vision for us, our Creator highly values each of us. After all, God came down from order and harmony of the heavens into a disordered, cacophonous creation, incarnate in Jesus, just for us. That is a statement of our worth in God's eyes. Wow!

DOES THE SOUL SLEEP IN DEATH?

Does the spirit or soul *sleep* at death, as some Biblical scholars suggest? Since this remains of mystery of our faith, I want to provide you with several perspectives on this idea of soul-sleep; be forewarned.

There are numerous scriptural passages proposing both a sleeping *material* and sleeping *immaterial* component for our being at death. We have Jesus' own words to Jairus, the Galilean synagogue ruler upon his daughter's death, "The child is not dead but asleep," (Mark 5:39); and friends and family of Lazarus' at Bethany. (John 11:1-44) "Our friend Lazarus has fallen asleep; but I am going there to wake him up." (John 11:11)

There are at least 36 references in the Scriptures that describe death as *sleep*. In fact, until late in the fifth century, this was the predominant teaching of the early Church.[120] Although subsequent theologians, including Augustine, move toward a teaching of an immortal soul, the reformer Luther returns to this original and Biblical concept of death as he writes, "It is probable, in my opinion, that, with very few exceptions indeed, the dead sleep in utter insensibility till the day of judgement....On what authority can it be said that the souls of the dead may not sleep...in the same way that the living pass in profound slumber the interval between their downlying at night and their uprising in the morning."[121,122] Yet this concept was not fully embraced by all in the Reformation, and actually not consistently by Luther himself.[123]

There are two Greek words for *sleep* in the New Testament. *Katheudo* is used 22 times and is used to describe naturally occurring sleep. The only time *katheudo* appears to be used to describe death is in the story of the raising of Jairus' daughter. In this setting, Jesus was saying that the grieving of the mourners was inappropriate and that their sadness would be shortly unnecessary as Jesus would raise the little girl from death.

On the other hand, the word *koimaomai* is used 18 times, and while it occasionally refers to natural sleep, 15 of the 18 times it is used to describe death as sleep.

The early Christians even referred to their burial grounds a *koimeteria,* "sleeping places," and this word is the root of our modern term for *cemetery.*

Let us return to the story of Lazarus. (John 11) John reports on this close family friend of Jesus from the town of Bethany who has fallen quite ill. Jesus decides to go to visit him, but he clearly understands this is a *teachable moment,* a time to glorify his Father. Jesus does not go until Lazarus has died, much to the chagrin of Lazarus' sisters (and Jesus' close friends) Mary and Martha. Jesus discusses Lazarus' condition with his disciples. He tells them Lazarus is *asleep* and he, Jesus, is going to *awaken* him. Hearing this, perhaps the disciples think that sleep is a good thing, it should help heal Lazarus.

But Jesus clarifies the condition. "Lazarus is dead," Jesus clearly states. Jesus emphatically tells his friends Lazarus is dead, not in *natural sleep,* and "I am glad I was not there, so that you may believe."

To Lazarus' grieving sister (again, a teachable moment), "I am the resurrection and the life. The one who believes in me will live, even though they die; and whoever lives by believing in me will never die. Do you believe this?"

Jesus awakens his friend as he, "Called in a loud voice, 'Lazarus, come out!'" Out comes Lazarus bound hand and foot in grave clothes. "Take off the grave clothes and let him go!"

Lazarus is not described as going to heaven or hell at the point of death, but entombed in sleep until he is "awakened" by a resurrection. So we have this instruction from the Lord on death.

As clear as any other passage in the Scriptures, Paul addresses this issue of what happens to those who die in Christ, those who believe in Christ as their Savior and Redeemer. In 1 Thessalonians 4:13-18, St. Paul refers to the righteous dead as being *asleep:*

> *"Brothers and sisters, we do not want you to be uniformed about those who <u>sleep</u> in death, so that you do not grieve like the rest of mankind, who have no hope. For we believe that Jesus died and rose again, and so we believe that God will bring with Jesus those who have <u>fallen asleep</u> in him. According to the Lord's word, we tell you that we who are still alive, who are left until the coming of the Lord, will certainly <u>not precede</u> those who have <u>fallen asleep</u>. For the Lord himself will come down from heaven, with a loud command, with the voice of the archangel and with the trumpet call of God, and the dead in Christ will rise first. After that, we who are still alive and are left will be caught up together with them in the clouds to meet the Lord in the air. And so we will be with the Lord forever. Therefore encourage one another with these words."*[124,125]

An Opposing View

In opposition, there are theologians and denominations who do not believe the soul is asleep or, for that matter, unconscious at the point of death. Rather, they teach that the body and soul separate at death, with the body sleeping in the grave, while the conscious soul departs and goes to live with Jesus or goes to a temporary holding zone (limbo or purgatory).

Supporting this thesis, the New Testament theologian D. Edmond Hiebert writes:

> "The figure of death as sleep cannot be pressed to establish the teaching that in the intermediate state the soul is in unconscious repose (soul sleep) ... the body only is thought of as being asleep, no longer in communication with its earthly environment. As sleep has its awakening, so the body of the believer will have its

awakening." Hiebert feels that soul sleep is inconsistent with Paul's assertion in 1 Thessalonians 5:10 that God's purpose for us is whether we live or die we should live together with Christ. I find *no* inconsistency with soul sleep in this passage:

"He died for us so that, whether we are awake or asleep, we may live together with him."

I believe that passage simply says that those who believe in Christ are *in* Christ whether physically dead or alive.

At death the believer's "earthly house or our tabernacle" is destroyed (2 Corinthians 5:1) and returns to the dust, but the spiritual part of man (and remember how Paul uses this term *spiritual as pneuma),* remains at *home* with the Lord. (2 Corinthians 5:8). Once again, Paul reminds us that to depart from the world in death and to "be with Christ, which is better by far" (Philippians 1:23) than the present state of being corruptible. Theologians like Hiebert argue, however, that "sleep" as applied to believers cannot be intended to teach that the soul is unconscious.[126]

Several theologians point out a few Biblical stories that would suggest at least some people's souls are alive or conscious after death. These stories include:

- Poor Lazarus and the rich man (Luke 16:19), and although meant as a *parable*, both Lazarus and Abraham are named as being in conversation in heaven.

- In the Transfiguration (Luke 9:30-31), Moses and Elijah appear with Jesus and appear quite *conscious.* However, the Transfiguration is not really about the *status* of Moses and Elijah but is about *Jesus.*

- Finally, on the Cross with the two thieves, Jesus promises the penitent robber, "Today you will be with me in Paradise." (Luke 23:43)[127]

The Teaching of the Immortality of the Soul as Being Dangerous

There are theologians (spiritists, they might be called) who argue that teaching a doctrine of an *immortal soul* is far more than a minor doctrinal issue but that it is a dangerous teaching. Some go as far as to call teaching that the soul is immortal may be one of Satan's greatest deceptions. They begin by pointing out Genesis 3:4:

> *"'You will not certainly die,' the serpent said to the woman."*

Or 2 Thessalonians 2:9-12:

> *"The coming of the lawless one will be in accordance with how Satan works. He will use all sorts of displays of power through signs and wonders that serve the lie, and all the ways that wickedness deceives those who are perishing. They perish because they refused to love the truth and so be saved. For this reason God sends them a powerful delusion so that they will believe the lie and so that all will be condemned who have not believed the truth but have delighted in wickedness."*

In this perspective on the soul at death, supporting theologians say Satan uses this idea of *familiar* or even *family spirits* (humans communicating from the grave) to again deceive us, and to deceive us with the same lie that Satan used to entrap Eve. Again, a few Old Testament passages speak to this lie and speak rather strongly:

> *"A man or woman who is a medium or spiritist among you must be put to death. You are to stone them; their blood will be on their own heads."* Leviticus 20:27

King of Israel, Saul, being challenged by the Philistine army, is calling on the Lord in fear, and not receiving dreams or prophetic response, seeks mediums instead of having faith in God. Saul asks the medium to speak to the deceased Samuel:

"Find me a woman, so I may go and inquire of her..." 1 Samuel 28:7

The medium says Samuel is speaking through her and that Samuel warns Saul of his demise along with his sons and army. And that is exactly what transpires in the remainder of 1 and 2 Samuel. God prefers faith; Saul's death should stand as a dire warning about how God feels about communicating with the dead.

To this point, the reformer Luther addresses the issue of "wandering souls" of the departed in purgatory. Luther strongly rejects the idea that "departed souls returned to plague the living with appeals for masses, vigils, and other services that would speed the wandering soul's movement out of purgatory."[128] Rather than being concerned about whether there was such a thing as "wandering souls", Luther's concern is that these souls should not distract the living from relying entirely on God's grace.[129, 130, 131]

Much of this discussion on mortal vs. immortal souls is addressed under the topic of a suspended or transitional location for the soul between death and the last Judgment. There are major efforts during the Protestant Reformation to address this topic and the historical power afforded the priesthood and work by loved ones in altering the length of transitioning, even to this day. Rather than addressing *transitioning* here, please visit the appendix to review a bit more on the topic of purgatory and limbo.

Soul-Sleep in Conclusion

Let me offer a contemporary perspective on soul-sleep from Rev. Dr. Jeff Gibbs, Professor of Exegetical Theology at Concordia Seminary, St. Louis. He contends that we can speak of the importance of the creedal statement regarding the resurrection of the body and the *nephesh-spirit* created as a whole being by God through describing what happens to us at death as *sleep,* but better yet as *rest and awaiting Christ.* Death is a *rest point* for the wholeness of corrupted mankind and a corrupted creation, and the next moment is the return of Christ to judge the world.

What are the practical quandaries of this debate regarding soul-sleep? Soul-disposition at death can be an extremely challenging discussion with grieving family, notes Dr. Kolb. "And I cannot imagine (as a pastor) how 'Isn't it nice that Charlie is sleeping in the cemetery rather than being at the supper table with you and the children' actually works at the funeral." I suspect you have overheard or joined a conversation containing sentiments of, "Well, at least mother is looking down on us approving (or disapproving) of each decision we make...."

Perhaps, says Dr. Gibbs, it is more helpful and Biblical to say, the soul (whole being) *"rests* at death, *awaiting* the return of Christ to restore all of creation."[132]

In summary, *soul-sleep,* whether conscious or unconscious at death, still remains a mystery, and may be a rather incomplete expression of what happens to us when we die. There remain some who insist that the ethereal nature of humankind immediately departs from the body, but disagree as to whether that nature is conscious or in a suspended state of consciousness? Or, as some faiths teach, the ethereal nature journeys to a temporary sidetrack, a place to work off some of the misdeeds of life, or may have others assist in the movement to union with God, i.e., a purgatory/limbo/ interim state. Or, finally, others insist the whole soul or ethereal nature journeys in time and space to inhabit a new cabinet, a new vessel, a new human or animal being, as is postulated in forms of reincarnation. This last teaching is not common in the Christian faith community, but is in other world religions.

As a follower of Christ (and I know I am sounding like a broken record) we do understand this:

At death, we will be with God, joined with God in inconceivable joy, eternally. With this still a magnificent mystery, some might find comfort in the way Dr. Kolb eloquently describes it: "I will spring from time into post-time/eternity and therefore *experience* the resurrection of the body, although transformed, immediately. As Christ promised the associate-crucified on the crosses of Calvary, 'Truly I tell you, today *you* will be with me in paradise.'" (Luke 23:43) The container, the material body, will go on to be altered whether by the oven or the oxygenation and bacteria-disintegration of the flesh, bones, and organs, and compacted or scattered, to be gathered and restored incorruptibly at the Last Judgment.

The Scriptures do assure us of this last promise from our Creator: there *will be* a day of Judgment for all the earth. The dead will be awakened and arise (wholly) before those still alive on that day. (1 Thessalonians 4:15) We don't know the day or the hour. We do know the judge—Christ. Those who believe in Jesus will be saved (an indescribable joy); those who do not will be damned. That's not good; way not good.

What will joyful life be like in heaven—or the dreadful existence in hell, for that matter? Not sure, is the best answer once again, even with the insight of some Biblical verses and scores of theological writings. The book of Revelation offers apocryphal (things hidden) descriptions of life in the hereafter, and I invite you to explore that book perhaps with some wonderful reading guides by authoritative authors like Rev. Dr. Louis Brighton, *Concordia Commentary: Revelation*, Concordia Publishing House, St. Louis, 1999.[133]

What we can know without question (because we are told so in God's Word) is that God is loving, so loving that God sent the Christ from the splendor of heaven into the pain of earth, and even into the depths of hell, in our place so that we could be with the Creator into eternity. God has the plan; God has the vision; God provides the pathway in Jesus. Jesus is preparing the way and the destiny (John 14:2-4), even as I am aging.

Ecclesiastes 9:5-10. "For the living know that they will die; but the dead know nothing...For there is no work or device or knowledge or wisdom in the grave where you are going."

Psalm 90:3-6. "You turn man back to dust and say, 'Return, O children of men.' For a thousand years in Your sight are like yesterday when it passes by, or as a watch in the night. You have swept them away like a flood, they fall asleep; in the morning they are like grass which sprouts anew."

Psalm 13:3. "Consider, and answer me, O Lord my God; enlighten my eyes, or I will sleep the sleep of death."

Daniel 12:2. The dead are "those who sleep in the dust of the earth," who shall "later awake" through being resurrected.

Job 3:11-17. "Why did I not die at birth? Why did I not die when I came from the womb...For now I would have lain still and been quiet, I would have been asleep; then I would have been at rest...There the wicked cease from troubling, and there the weary are at rest."

1 Kings 11:43. "And Solomon slept with his fathers and was buried in the city of his father David."

"Slept with his fathers," is the exact term referring to many of the kings of Israel to describe their death throughout 1 and 2 Kings.

Matthew 9:24, from the story of Jarius' daughter. Jesus admonishes the mourners and says, "Leave; for the girl has not died, but is asleep."

Mark 5:39, the same story is reported. "Why make a commotion and weep? The child has not died, but is asleep."

And just for emphasis, Luke reports the conversation of Jesus regarding Jairus' daughter. "Stop weeping, for she has not died, but is asleep."

WHAT HAPPENS TO THE SOUL AT DEATH?
A DISCUSSION OF PURGATORY AND GRACE

In medieval theology and the traditional teachings of the Roman Catholic Church, a purgatory served to "work off" the sins of temporal life so that those destined for heaven could undergo purification so as to achieve their holiness. Everyone in purgatory was eventually destined for heaven. The priest, giving the absolution of your sins, had the power to forgive original or so-called "mortal sin." The priest then assigned *activities of faith* to atone for temporal sins while you were yet alive. But at death, there remained sins that you had not atoned for in life. For these "venial sins," you proceeded to an interim state to "work off" the sin either by yourself, or with the help atonement-activities performed by your living loved ones. These activities atoned for sins that "stuck on to your account" so to speak.

Limbo was a concept developed in the Middle Ages, and not necessarily a part of Roman Catholic doctrine, that described a speculation on the afterlife of those who died and whose souls were barred from heaven but not yet consigned to Hell. There was a *limbus partum* (the Old Testament place where saints where thought to be confined until they were liberated by Christ in his descent into hell). There was also a *limbus infantum* (children's or infantile limbo) for those who die without actual sinning, but whose original sin had not been cleansed yet by baptism or who had been mentally deficient so that they could not exercise free will.[134] Contemporary Roman Catholic theology has a much more benevolent doctrine on the topic of infant death prior to baptism, and limbo plays little role.

So there remains a divide within religious communities as to the reality of a place in between earth and eternity, whether the final disposition is heaven or hell. For those who define their core identity via their own performance in life rather than by their grace-filled relationship with a merciful and loving Creator, a *purgatory-concept* becomes strategic, and in fact, essential for hope. If you believe your performance (your good or bad works) determines, in the end, what really counts in restoring your favor with God, you might value a purgatory. Whether those works must be performed while you are yet alive or can also be retrofitted by deeds in the afterlife by you or others on your behalf, a purgatory may have a place in your theology.

If, on the other hand, you believe that once restored in baptism into Christ, you cannot fall beyond God's grip of grace, despite your inadequacies, that there is only one atonement for your sin (and that being Christ alone), then a purgatory is of little to no use.

That term *grace* then needs clarification. In the middle ages of the Church, that term *grace* meant the instillation of a power from God to perform good works, to reconnect as a disordered, relationally disconnected human being with our Creator by our own deeds. In the Protestant Reformation of the 1500s, through the writings of reformers like Luther and based on understanding of Hebrew (Old Testament) and Greek (New Testament) writings, *grace* becomes understood as God's *favor*, God's *unwavering love and mercy* toward us. Here again, the soul/spirit *trusts* that we have been made whole, righteous, restored to relationship through Christ's life and death and resurrection. We understand ourselves as now being righteous (passively) and act accordingly (actively). "We agree (fear, love, trust) with God; we just do it," states the previously referenced Rev. Dr. Robert Kolb.

How does this happen (psychologically), you might ask? Dr. Kolb continues, "It is in the mystery of the gift of grace, is the best answer I know. How do we learn to trust, or for that matter love another human being, a spouse or a child for example. Well, I suppose some of trust and love come out of their consistent faithfulness toward us. If their love in unwavering, there response to our need consistent (as humanly possible), we learn to trust them. Love may be a bit more mysterious. *Eros,* romantic love, or even *philia,* fellowship, may involve all sorts of biochemical and biophysical sequelae of sight, and sound, and smell, and experience. But *agape,* unconditional love, comes from faithfulness and commitment." God is faithful and committed to us through Christ.[135]

WHAT DOES CHRISTIAN THEOLOGY TEACH REGARDING DUALISM? UNDERSTANDING A SEPARATE BODY AND MIND/ SOUL VS. MONISM (INSEPARABLE BODY AND MIND/SOUL)

One way to map out Genesis 2:7 is with the following equation: *body + God's spirit = soul*. It is not without its challengers, even in traditional doctrinal teachings. I want to touch on that issue once more. Sadly, and in disservice to the Church, as I will discuss in the following paragraphs, the *dualism* (separated entities of body and mind/soul/spirit deeply imbedded in Greek thought), influences traditional and confessional writings of some theologians and Church leaders. In fact, dualism is gradually moved by ecclesiastical and historical tradition in the Church toward the teaching of purgatory as noted above. Church tradition fuels *dualism* with a priesthood given powerful authority to administer sacraments and dole out indulgences to, in essence, buy the soul's way out of a prolonged time of penance in purgatory.

The Protestant Reformers begin to address the sequelae of dualism of mankind in church teachings in the early 1500s. But a century later dualism was reinforced by Descartes (1600s), from which we may only now be emerging.

Please allow me an additional comment on soul and spirit. Both soul and spirit might be considered *mortal* or *immortal*, depending on the doctrinal belief system.[136] In some Judaic and Christian denominations all living organisms have souls, but only humans have *immortal* souls. In other denominations, humans but not animals are considered to be possessors of souls. Religions like Jainism and Hinduism attribute souls to all living organisms, and other religions like animism believe that *all* things possess souls, even rivers and mountains.

In contemporary Christian theology we often see teaching that when a person dies, they immediately go to their everlasting dwelling (proceed outside of the limits of time), either heaven or hell. This has raised the subsequent question of what then would be the purpose of a Judgment Day or Final Judgment that is clearly described in the Scriptures. Human death, incidentally, is a horrible, horrible happening—the worst consequence of sin. Even though we say for people having pain from cancer or immobility from neurologic disease, that it brings sweet relief (and it does), death is still a horrid event.

Consider these directives:

> "...But man dies and is laid away; Indeed he breathes his last And where is he?
>
> As water disappears from the sea, And a river becomes parched and dries up, so man lies down and does not rise. Till the heavens are no more, They will not awake Nor be roused from their sleep." (Job 14:10-12 KJV)
>
> "...Do not marvel at this; for the hour is coming in which all who are in the graves will hear His voice and come forth-those who have done good, to the resurrection of life, and those who have done evil, to the resurrection of condemnation."
>
> (John 5:28,29 KJV)
>
> "...Men and brethren, let me speak freely to you of the patriarch David, that he is both dead and buried, and his tomb is with us to this day... For David did not ascend into the heavens." (Acts 2:29, 34 KJV)
>
> "...Behold, I tell you a mystery: We shall not all sleep, but we shall all be changed in a moment, in the twinkling of an eye, at the last trumpet. For the trumpet will sound, and the dead will be raised incorruptible, and we shall be changed." (1 Corinthians 15:51, 52 KJV)

These passages suggest that mankind ceases to function (is fully mortal) and sleeps or at least *rests* in death, and *awaits* the Resurrection, some to everlasting life with God, and some to everlasting separation from God (damnation).

But what about Christ's words to his cross-mate; does that provide both clarity an assurance?

"Today, you will be with me in paradise." (Luke 23:43) This certainly assures us that Christ's redemption has been accomplished on the Cross, once and for all time.

Further, consider Paul's address to the Corinthians: *"We are confident, I say, and would prefer to be away from the body and at home with the Lord."* (2 Corinthians 5:8) *"...So we are always confident, knowing that while we are at home in the body we are absent from the Lord for we walk by faith, not by sight. We are confident, yes, well pleased rather to be absent from the body and to be present with the Lord."* (2 Corinthians 5:6-8)

Do these passages, on the other hand, suggest that natures of humankind separate with the body resting in the grave and the soul or spirit dwelling with Christ? Are the natures only reunited at the Last Judgment? The best answer is, "I don't know."

Dualism of the Soul and Spirit in the Early Church

St. Paul begins to address the beliefs and applications of both Greek and Jewish thoughts on dualism of soul/spirit and body in his Epistles to the early churches in Asia.

St. Paul, schooled in Greek philosophy and thinking, undoubtedly has been taught that the human soul has three interrelated elements: a body or material component with desires and drives; a mind or cognitive component with thoughts, memory, perceptions, and responses that also knows the difference between good and evil but not always being able to influence the body; and finally, an organizing principle or a spirit, all of which incorporate the whole being or soul. And yet, I think we hear Paul's letters exclaim, we do not *have* a soul, we *are* a soul; we do not *have* a body, we *are* a body. Is this a more *monistic* theology, perhaps? Look further at how Paul uses the term *soul*.

One example of this use of *soul* is in Paul's writings in 1 Corinthians 15, contrasting Adam and Christ. Referring to Genesis 2, Paul says Adam (the first Adam) was created as a living *soul* (nephesh—living, breathing organism). So Adam *is* a psyche/soul; he doesn't just have a *soul*. But the soul-Adam is *mortal*. Christ (the last Adam), on the other hand, was raised as a life-giving Spirit. Therefore the resurrected Christ has the potential to impart the same eternal life to us, as we daily live a new life on our earthy journey, and into the future when, additionally, our disordered and diseased bodies can be redeemed and made incorruptible or clean—whole beings.

However, the Greek-trained Paul expresses real concerns about the reliance on Greek philosophy and household codes of living creeping into some of the early Christian faith communities in Asia Minor. He addresses these concerns specifically to the Church in Colossae, a small Phrygian city about 100 miles from Ephesus, and the Ephesians themselves. The Colossians appear to be incorporating pagan elements into their daily life-practice (men's' authority over wives, children, and slaves, for example), and are worshiping elemental spirits, as do the Greeks. (Colossians 3:12-4:6) Paul exhorts Christ's supremacy over all of creation, and that Christ alone is the intermediary to God, the very agent of reconciliation and salvation. (Colossians 1:20) He reminds the Colossians not to trust on other philosophies and traditions that do not depend on Christ alone.

Paul's letters stand in contrast to Aristotle's "Greek" household codes, found in his *Politics,* and followed in many homes through Asia Minor in order to keep *Pax Romana*.[137] Paul reminds all the faith communities of the early Church that Jesus adds a new element to not just the contemporary theology of the day, but that Jesus changes *everything*. Jesus is now the master of the family and household, but he rules and organizes the home through humility and love rather than legalism.

St. Paul also contrasts with the anthropologic dualism of Plato (we have a body that is human, material, mortal, and of the world, *and* we have a separate soul or mind that is eternal, the true person, and divine). One might deduce that Paul is suggesting *dualism* with his address of *flesh* and *spirit.* However, Paul uses the word *flesh* to describe the power of corruption in the world and human life, rather than the body *per se.* In contrast, Paul uses the word *spirit* for the capacity of God to transform our lives, including our bodies, both now and at the resurrection. *Flesh* and *spirit* are contrasting powers that can affect every dimension of life, rather than two components of the human person. For St. Paul, flesh is the corrupted world; spirit is the way of Christ.

Paul never contrasts *soul* or *psyche* to the *body.* He really doesn't think of a human as body separate from soul; his use of these terms *soul* or *soulish* (psychikos) are as *value-laden* terms.

In this *value-laden* sense, St. Paul describes how our *soul* is organized, identifying what he calls the Spirit as the re-organizing principle within our being as exemplified in 1 Corinthians 2:14-15: He uses two Greek terms:

Psychikos: soul or *soulish;* the natural man, as a rather pathetic effort of a soul separated from God due to sin and trying to organize itself. The direction of the soul's energy is disordered, unhealthily directed inward = *ME.* You are on your own, so you better be anxious and directed to looking out for ME.

Pneumatikos: Spirit-directed; the way God intended the soul to be organized by the power of God's Holy Spirit. The direction of the soul's energy is enlivened, empowered, transformed, non-anxious, and focused outward into loving relationships = *WE.* We with God, we with our neighbor, we in harmony with all of creation.

Christ's Spirit witnesses to our sinful, inwardly focused soul (psychikos) and heals our damaged being, reorganizing our entire being so that our energy flows now outward to fearing, loving, and trusting God and into service of God and God's creation. Rather than living alone, isolated, and separate, one now is living resiliently and abundantly in communion with God. (1 Corinthians 15)

Does Paul address *salvation* of the soul or spirit? *Salvation* of the *soul* or *soulish-ness* is addressed by other Epistle writers (1 Peter 1:1-9; Hebrews 10:39) referring to *soul* meaning the *whole person*, but not by St. Paul who doesn't see *soul* as *just one part* of the person. Again, Paul sees the human *soul* as the corrupt world passing away thanks to Christ alone.

As the Church moves across the earth in time, *mortality* vs. *immortality* of the *soul* come up again in the third to fifth centuries. There is a controversy among theologians in three areas of this belief: the Universalists do not believe in an everlasting Hell; the Conditionalists support the idea of sleep of body and soul at death; and the Immortal Soulists believe that the soul ascends to God at human death. These controversies serve as dividing points in the first millennium of the Church.

In the 1200s, Thomas Aquinas reiterates Greek philosophy, especially Aristotle's contention that the soul is the first *actuality* of life and that there are three types of living beings: plants that feed and grow; animals that bring the addition of sensation to plants; and humans that provide intellect to the activity of animals. Aquinas reasons that the soul does not have to rely on a body to exist since the soul is incorporeal. Therefore the soul also cannot be destroyed by any natural process.[138]

Then, beginning with Martin Luther in Germany and William Tyndale in England, the long-buried concept of the *sleep* or *rest* of humankind in death, and the awakening at the Resurrection, gathers adherents which surfaces from the Reformation to modern times.

Martin Luther and other 16th-century reformers were reacting to the papal traditional and authoritative teachings including an unending Hell and a purifying purgatory, and the matter of the consciousness of the soul in death. Luther and Tyndale prefer to return to the pre-fourth-century Church writings, early Apostolic thoughts, and most importantly, the original Holy Scriptures themselves.

In breaking with the papacy and in his scriptural-based stand of faith at the Diet of Worms, Luther becomes a national voice for reforms of many of the practices instilled in the medieval Roman Catholic Church. Luther's writings on justification by faith become a keystone of the Reformation. More about justification as it pertains to this discussion in a moment. His translation of the Bible from Latin into German make him a leader in the German tongue of expression and restores the reading and study of the Scriptures to the common man.

Luther carefully confronts unscriptural positions that have come into common acceptance, and coincidentally elevate the power of the priesthood and the papacy. In particular, Luther examines the teachings of the immortality of the soul and the consciousness of the soul in death during the pains of purgatory. Much of his thought is based on his reading of a complete copy of the Latin Bible while he was studying law at the University of Erfurt.

The ecclesiastical focus of the Middle Ages is the instilling of fear of God in the people to bolster unquestioning reverence to the Church and the papacy. Luther, confined to a monastery in the early 1500s, serves his time in penance and study of the Scriptures. Monastically, he is seeking the forgiveness of his sins, his salvation, through the penitential system—a righteousness "through good works" approach to gaining God's favor.

Luther has learned well the dominant medieval themes of trying to escape the horrors of Hell through living a life of piety. Purgatory is a concept introduced to mitigate the length of time and intensity of punishment between death and the Last Judgment through the use of penances, purchase of indulgences (*get out of jail papers*), praying to saints for intercession, and the Church offering her sacraments.

Based on his reading of Scripture, Luther rejects the Church's teachings of a predestined fate of consignment to Hell or Heaven for a soul from creation, turning instead to a teaching of hope from a loving God. Again, now as a Doctor of Divinity and professor of the Scriptures at the University of Wittenberg, and a profound, Latin, Greek and Hebrew scholar, Luther questions all teachings and traditions of the Church in the face of what was written directly in the Bible. A penultimate Scriptural message Luther believes is that salvation and restoration to God's family comes through Christ's substitutionary death on the Cross and his Resurrection. For Luther, this is the message of the Gospel pure and simple.

For emphasis, the Gospel message proclaimed by the Reformation and found in St. Paul's writings consists of these foundational tenets:

- Redemption comes from faith in Christ, not from human effort. Salvation is a gift, not a result of penance summarized in the phrase, "*Word alone; Faith alone; Grace alone.*" (*Sola scriptura; Solo fide; Sol gratia*) This phrase states the Scripture presides over tradition; faith over works; grace over merit.

- Truth is found in the Holy Scriptures alone as the inerrant communication of God to creation.

- We are justified, made right with God, by faith in Christ alone (Solus Christus). Living a good life is a sign of faith, not a prerequisite for salvation.

Let me just define this term *justification* just a bit more as it pertains to the disposition of the soul and spirit. Justification, in Christian theology, means God's act of removing the guilt and penalty of sin while simultaneously declaring a sinful person righteous through Christ's atoning substitution on the Cross in our stead.

The true distinction, therefore, between the Protestant (certainly Lutheran and Calvinism) and the Roman Catholic view of *justification* is not an issue of being "declared righteous" versus being "made righteous," but rather it is the *means* by which one is justified. In Catholic theology righteous works are considered meritorious toward salvation *in addition* to faith; whereas in most Protestant theology, righteous works are seen as the *result and evidence* of a truly justified and regenerate believer who has received these by faith alone."[139]

Furthermore, Luther writes in 1520 a published Defense of 41 of his 95 theses posted on the Wittenberg Church door (the academic bulletin board of the day) in 1517. He specifically challenges the teaching that the soul is immortal. Luther, rather, espouses a *sleep* of the soul in death, and does so upon a Scriptural foundation. He uses this to counter the teachings of purgatory (a conscience torment of the soul in death) and worshiping and petitioning of saints. Luther asserts that Scripture teaches that the soul is at rest, asleep, awaiting the second coming of Christ in death; not conscious, not aware.[140, 141] At the resurrection, our body and soul are awakened from this sweet sleep and come alive to meet our Savior.

Luther is writing before Descartes. Descartes strongly proposes dualism as a way we can *scientifically understand* functions of body and spirit, in the setting of the teachings of the Church. It is, says Descartes, better to understand man as a unified yet dual body-soul entity and he defends this as more Biblical.[142]

Descartes provides a saying summing up this dualism concept, "cognito ergo sum," or "I reflect therefore I am." In saying this, Descartes returns to the notion that the immaterial mind and the material body are two completely different substances, although they interact with each other. Incidentally, Descartes teaches essentially that the terms "mind" and the "soul" are the same thing.

The teachings of Descartes do have some value to the progress of science; they allow the scientific community to begin to explore the physical world, as the Church prohibited science from touching anything *divine*. The mind is seen as God's realm; the body then is totally a separate and non-divine entity, and not part of God's divine image. It is worth noting that modern "string theory" and "Higgs boson" actually suggest a breaking down of this duality as everything is seen as merely forms of *energy*.

As a believer of Jesus as our Savior, I think we can be confident that at death we are *with* Jesus. How does that work exactly, being a creature living in the constraints of time? Are we in a suspended or interim state until the Last Judgment? Are we conscious, aware, thinking? I don't think we know.

I do know this about those of faith in Christ at death, and I believe it is a truth of great comfort: we are without pain and suffering; we are at peace, not anxious; we are at rest, not struggling; we are eagerly anticipating and awaiting Jesus' return to finally heal all that is creation. I don't believe it is critical, even as a scientifically trained physician, to have perfect clarity of all those details, but it is critical to have that assurance. We do!

WHAT DOES JESUS TELL US ABOUT THE SOUL? THE CONTEXT OF JESUS' MINISTRY, AGING AND HIS END OF LIFE TEACHINGS

Preceding the time of Christ, many religions and philosophies were wrestling with the idea of soul and spirit.

Just before Christ's birth, the Athenian school of Greek philosophers—Socrates, Plato, and Aristotle—all developed descriptions and definitions of soul-ness, perhaps out of a longing for more than earthly confines. I alluded to these earlier in the appendix. We also looked at some of the ancient teachings on humanness and soul in Egypt, China, and India in the appendix. Suffice it to say that Christ comes down from the heavens into an Asia Minor and Major inundated with a variety of thoughts and teachings on the soul.

At the same time and in roughly the same geography, Hebrew Scripture forms the foundation for Hebrew theological sects, like the Sadducees and the Pharisees who are wrestling with the idea of the soul as Jesus appears.

The writers of the Torah use the terms *nephesh* (vital breath or life) and *ruach* (spirit) in the first chapter of Genesis to describe *soul*.

The Sadducees were an aristocratic, wealthy, and politically powerful majority in the ruling council or Sanhedrin. They included many chief priests and the high priest. They were working hard at keeping the peace with their Roman occupiers, and it would be fair to say they may have been more concerned with the political rather than religious rulings of the day. They tended to associate with the upper class supporters than with the common Israeli citizen.

The Sadducees were doctrinally conservative, considering only the written Word of God to be authoritatively from God (the first five books of the Old Testament—Genesis through Deuteronomy). Of particular interest to this discussion, the Sadducees denied any resurrection of the dead including the accounts of Christ. (Matthew 22:23; Mark 12:18-27; Acts 23:8) They rejected any idea of the afterlife, holding that the *soul* perished at death; therefore there was no reward of punishment after earthly life. They did believe, however, in the existence of a spiritual world filled with angels and demons.

The Sadducees were really not concerned about Jesus until Christ began to attract Roman attention and appeared as a threat to their *kingdom*. At that point they colluded with the Pharisees to bring Christ to crucifixion. They persecuted others of Jesus' Apostles and family. The Sadducees were ousted from power when Rome destroyed Jerusalem and the temple in 70 CE.

The Pharisees, on the other hand, were the middle-class businessmen and allied with the working class of Israel. Being supported by the common man, they held substantial power within the Sanhedrin. They also held the written Word as inspired by God, but they also gave equal weight to the oral tradition that they believe extended all the way back to Moses. These oral traditions, which fill out the remainder of the Old Testament, were held by the Pharisees as equal to God's Word and we see this struggle addressed by the early Christian Church in numerous examples. (Matthew 9:14; 15:1-9; 23:5; Mark 7:1-23; Luke 11:42)

Pharisees did believe in the resurrection of the dead (Acts 23:6) and an afterlife associated with appropriate reward and punishment. They concurred with the Sadducees on the reality of angels and demons. They also collaborated with the Sadducees, as noted, to put Jesus to death (Mark 14:53; 15:1; John 11:48-50)

The Pharisees actually exist post the destruction of Jerusalem by Rome and are instrumental in the continuation of Judaism beyond the destruction of the temple in 70 CE.

In the Christian faith, we disagree with the teachings of the Sadducees by believing all that is held in the Scriptures (even beyond Genesis to Deuteronomy) as the Word of God, and the continuation of life after death. And unlike the Pharisees, we are *not* to treat *traditions* as having equal authority to God's Word, nor are we to allow our relationship with God to be reduced to the *legalism* of rules and rituals. That is a lesson we need to hear from the Lord within our Christian faith again today.

Certainly, some of these *soul-issues* and *kingdom of God-issues* were contributory to the conflicts addressed by Jesus throughout his ministry, and fuel some of the anger, anxieties, and agitation that eventually drive nails through his hands and feet into the Cross.

Nonetheless, the reason for Jesus' birth, walk, death, and resurrection in our earthly midst was exactly to redeem our souls, our whole beings. And his promise is to return again to heal all of creation.

HOW DOES THE SOUL FIT INTO THE DOCTRINE OF LAW AND GOSPEL?

For those who wish a more in depth discussion of soul and spirit theology through the history of the Christian church, I would invite you to explore the appendix under Dualism of Body and Soul vs. the Soul as the Whole Being in Church Teachings. For others, there may be more interest in exploring a few more contemporary aspects on exploring the soul from a couple of additional avenues of theological thought.

A current resource for this topic is the afore-mentioned Rev. Dr. Robert Kolb. Asked directly, Professor Kolb addresses the subject of the soul rather succinctly: "I really do not know what the soul is."

With that underlying tenet, he goes on to explain that there are at least two great mysteries we wrestle with; how can there be a God who is three persons in one (the Trinity), and what does it mean to be human? The Scriptures (the words that God uses to reveal God being God and God sending to mankind a God-man Son) describe God as almighty and all-determinative. The Scriptures also describe humans as being made in God's image yet still responsible for the choices we make and the things we do. These positions of God and man would seem incongruent, and it remains for us beyond our ability to gather into one unifying concept.

Dr. Kolb suggests that a valuable venue to place these theological conundra is within the bewilderment we associate with the distinction of *law* and *gospel:* God gives all things but holds us responsible for being obedient to God's design for our lives—body, mind, and soul/spirit. God gives us *law,* in particular a set of ten laws or commandments, the first of which is that we humans are to *fear, love, and trust God in all things.* This means that we are to be faithful or faith-filled within a relationship in which God promises to be faithful to us—no matter what! However, that human-God relationship, at least from the human side, is tempered by the presence of *evil*, of *doubt*, of *sin*. Sin does not infect God, but is a formidable destructive power within our daily existence. "No biblical writer, however, explains the terms "soul" and "spirit" to us satisfactorily," states Dr. Kolb. The writers of the Scriptures always communicate to us about body, but some authors speak of just the *soul*, and others of *soul and spirit*.[143]

Contemporary theology continues to reference reformation writings that define *spirit* as the *relationship with the Creator*. Earlier we mentioned Luther's definition of *being human* beginning with our "fearing, loving, and trusting in God above all things"—First Commandment stuff. Today, as we think about what it is that God actually breathed into the human creation, we think of the capacity to "fear, love, and trust" in God above all, especially above trusting self.

Furthermore, God gifts the human soul not just with the capacity to love, but with the **gift of *being loved* unconditionally**. This very truth about the relationship breathed into God's human creation is stated as clearly as is possible in 1 John 4:10:

> "This is love: not that we loved God, but that He loved us and sent His Son as an atoning sacrifice for our sins."

Professor Kolb states, "He (Luther) had no doctrine of God as revealed (and we daresn't talk about his Hidden God, he says) apart from God's relationship to his creation, particularly to us human beings, and he (Luther) has no understanding of being human apart from centering our humanity on what we ultimately trust."[144]

While yet turned into ourselves, our whole being as humans is *governed* by the trust in God that Christ has created through his death for our sins in our stead and his resurrection to restore our identity as belonging solely to God, as being the Creator's beloved children.[145]

DOES THE SOUL AGE? THE THEOLOGY OF PASSIVE AND ACTIVE RIGHTEOUSNESS

It is within the context of the soul's disposition and destination that we might tackle the topic of whether or not the soul or spirit ages. We return to the known purposes of humankind to be in loving relationship with the Creator—to *know* God, to *fear, love, and trust* God. Christ's reconciliatory work on the Cross (breathed into us in our Baptismal* promise from God and, therefore, restoring that *relationship),* does not, cannot, and will not change. God is faithful. God's promise is sure. The promise and relationship that inform our whole being does not change, does not age.

*Note on Baptismal covenant: Although different meaning and purpose is given in various denominations to baptism, the shared significance is that baptism is a promise of God to God's followers to adopt them as God's own children. The covenant is received by us by water placed upon us but that water is included in God's command and combined with God's Word. It gives us the forgiveness of our sins. In other words, it is redemption or salvation and it is received by faith alone, that faith being the knowledge, acceptance of, and trust in the promise of Christ's saving and reconciliatory work of death in our place. Even faith itself is seen as an undeserved gift of God, created in the hearts of God's children by the work of the Holy Spirit through God's Word and Baptism.

What certainly may change, wax and wane, deteriorate or mature, is our feelings of fear, love, and trust in God, *especially in the face of* God's faithfulness to us. God is faithful to the *gift of relationship,* distinct from the gifts that flow to and from the relationship. *Our* psychological and spiritual aspects of perceiving our relationship with God may falter, due to our inward-focused self, a deteriorating flesh, and the efforts of Satan. In other words, *we* may periodically *doubt* God's faithfulness and promises in relationship to us when things don't go *"our way."* For example, even though we have been praying fervently for God to cure us of cancer, we may return to the doctor's office only to hear, "I'm afraid the cancer has returned in the lymph nodes."

Those of you who have dealt with chronic disease like cancer or addictions, mental illness, or devastating loss of loved ones, understand well how your whole being, including your sense of relationship with God, can be challenged. It is real and it is tempting to ask in these circumstances, "My God, my God, why have You forsaken me?" We can falter, we can doubt.

It is in the midst of this doubtfulness that it may be helpful and proper to divert to the theological topic of *justification and righteousness* before our Creator. Martin Luther coined the terms *passive righteousness* and *active righteousness.*[146] As we wrestle with relational doubt it may be helpful to people of any Christian faith to understand how we can be made and remain *right* or *justified* in our relationship with God, especially in the face of challenges of illness and eminent death.

Passive righteousness refers to our core identity (who we are and how God sees us), which is determined by Christ alone and established through Christ's atoning death in our stead. We experience and receive that righteousness through our faith and trust. *Active righteousness* is our *agreeing* with God that we are God's children and so our actions and stewardship behavior correspond through praising, loving, and serving God and the rest of God's creation. God's gift of passive righteousness through Christ does not change, even in aging, even in those demented or with dysfunctional and irrational moods and emotions, even in those with clouded minds and consciences, or those too young for extensive rational thought. Our *active righteousness* may well alter with aging. We may not steadily grow in the Spirit, tell the good news, steward wisely or faithfully as we get older; our perception of our purpose and mission may indeed grow or falter. That part of *soul-ness* may age. "We may truly suffer a weariness of the soul," suggests Dr. Kolb. What other writers might call "weariness" I would call "losing resilience of the soul."

Therefore our soul, defined by the relationship with our Creator, does not change or age because God's love for us through Christ does not change. Our appreciation and response to that loving relationship, our faithfulness to Christ, is continuously challenged by the evil forces of this world—Satan, the distresses, illnesses, disease, and death all part of this world, and our own inwardly focused desires. That appreciative, responsiveness may "age," be "less than resilient" along our life journey. Yet in God's Spirit through Christ, we are given the loving resources to renew our fear, love, and trust of God.

We are reminded of a "trustworthy saying," proclaimed in 2 Timothy 2:13:

> *"...if we are faithless, he remains faithful, for he cannot disown himself."*

That's a good enough promise for me, and I hope it is for you!

So to summarize the theology of soul and spirit we have dipped deeply into teachings of *both* law and Gospel and the doctrines of justification and righteousness. I believe a reasonable and faithful historical and contemporary answer to the question, "Does the soul age?" is the following:

> *The soul is the best word to encapsulate the immaterial and ethereal, God-created and gifted human nature we would call the spirit or breath of God, mysteriously united with the God-created and gifted physical human nature of dust (atoms and energy). A soul is unique to one individual, and exists from God's creative act of conception, and from that moment wholly encompasses what it means to be human. That human soul is loved by the Creator unconditionally and gifted with the capacity to love. It is made righteous in God's heart because of God's Son, Jesus Christ, who restores the harmony of the relationship lost because of sin. We receive this righteousness passively, not of our doing. In Christ, we are invited to actively participate in the stewarding these many gifts*

of God's love for us, to conform to God's good will for us, to live in agreement with God. We do not have clarity about the state of the soul at human death, but we have assurance of its disposition and destination at the Last Judgment of the earth and its inhabitants, especially for those who die in Christ—we will live wholly and eternally with God in light and joy.

Those are mind and imagination-straining sentences, right? Nevertheless, I believe they well-describe a Scriptural truth and frame a mystery of Christian faith. However, far better than reflecting on the feeble attempts of a 21st-century physician to describe being a human with and aging body, mind, and spirit, I remind you to turn and proclaim one of the great creeds of our faith: the **Apostle's Creed**, the **Nicene Creed** or the **Athanasian Creed**—they say it all.

IS THE SOUL UNIQUELY HUMAN?

Religious and philosophical communities vary as to what and who in the universe possess souls. There are even diverse teachings in Jewish and Christian traditions. I trust the Scriptural words that, "God formed the man from the dust of the ground and breathed into his nostrils the breath of life, and the man became a living being [soul]." (Genesis 2:7) Man was made and gifted separately from animals and the rest of creation. There is no Scriptural prohibition to the killing of animals (although it is to be done humanely), but there is to the killing of fellow humankind. "You shall not murder," speaks to our responsibilities to fellow humans. (Exodus 20:13) Furthermore, we know God demands animal sacrifice in the Old Testament and does give animals for human consumption until after the Flood in Genesis 9. For these reasons, I believe God has gifted souls only to human creatures.

WORD-SATURATED MEDITATIVE PRAYER

We live in a multi-tasking culture. Discourse and relationships are constantly under threat, especially our conversations with our Creator. Noise and hurry predominate over quiet and stillness. The Scriptures throughout, however, invite us to "pause" and "pivot." "Be still and know that I am God." (Psalm 46:10) Our God invites us to enter communication in this relationship with quiet, solitude, stillness, and deeply immersed in God's Word; in fact, saturated in the Word.

Yet we are threatened with noise and hurry, and the predictable sequelae of fear and anxiety. Noise: our environment is filled with auditory stimulation—TV, radio, Internet, YouTube, and Pandora, to name just a few. Frequently we are plugged in and tuned out. What may be worse is the cacophony of internal conversation that generally is filled with negative self-talk rather than positive self-hugs. Think about your last conversation with yourself. Was it characterized by, "God loves you and so do I," or was it filled with derogatory words like *idiot, stupid, dumbbell* or worse? We are good at making ourselves a terrific target for Satan to establish a base of operations within to try to separate us from each other and from our Savior.

And then there's hurry. Chief of sinners have I been in my life as a physician, husband, father, and friend. I love the quote of the Swiss counselor and analytical psychiatrist Carl Jung who said, "Hurry is not of the devil; it is the devil." (Paraphrasing St. Jerome's "*Omnis festinatio ex parte diabolic est*"—"All haste is of the devil.")

In contrast, we hear the story of Elijah as he is exhausted and depressed after being chased by Jezebel. (1 Kings 19:1-18) God calls Elijah to a time and a place of solitude, rest, restoration, and healing. The Creator comes to Elijah in a *whisper.*

Or we recall the story of Mary and Martha of Bethany. Martha (Type A) is busily cleaning the home and cooking the feast, and looking for her sister, Mary, who chooses to sit at the feet of the Master and *listen* ... (Luke 10:38-4)

Or, the Sermon on the Mount, when Jesus gives us the Lord's Prayer,

"And when you pray, do not be like the hypocrites; for they love to pray standing in the synagogues...to be seen by men... they have received their reward in full. But when you pray, go into your room, close the door and pray to your Father who is unseen...for your Father knows what you need before you ask him. Then this is how you should pray: 'Our Father in heaven...'" (Matthew 6:5-14)

Finally, based on the Scriptures and in the voice of the 16th-century reformer, Martin Luther's well-known Christmas hymn:

"Ah, dearest Jesus, holy Child,

Make thee a bed, soft, undefiled,

Within my heart that it may be,

A quiet chamber kept for thee."

Christ extends to us the invitation to pause, ponder, and pivot, especially in the setting of God's Word. The form of prayer we share on Grace Place Wellness Retreats (www.graceplacewellness.org) for clergy and educators follows the patterns of meditative, Word-focused prayer used throughout the history of the Church. More contemporary applications can be found under the catalogues of *Centering* or *Contemplative Prayer* (Fr. Thomas Keating), *Lectio Divina* (St. Augustine), or even in the *Oratio, Meditatio, Tentatio* suggested by Dr. Martin Luther. I will share with you our practice of Word-Saturated Meditative Prayer used on Grace Place Wellness Retreats.

There is value in setting aside time to saturate our prayer life in the Holy Scriptures and center our being in Christ by actually praying the Word of God, speaking in God's language, and aligning ourselves with God's will. This can be done in a quiet and unhurried setting.

These prayer disciplines call us back to mindfully spending time listening to and reflecting on what God self-reveals especially about the saving and substitutionary sacrifice of Jesus' cross, death, and resurrection. This prayer sets our intention on Christ in quiet, focused, supplicating, receiving, and thankful postures before God's throne of grace and mercy.

Our prayer follows the four-part circular, payer-pattern of *Lectio Divina*, and superimposes Luther's concept of *Oratio, Meditatio, and Tentatio* into a finite time frame for the purpose of praying "hours" of daily prayer (realizing that was not necessarily the specific intent of Luther's guidance to us).

Word-Saturated Meditation
QUIETING AND SLOWING DOWN

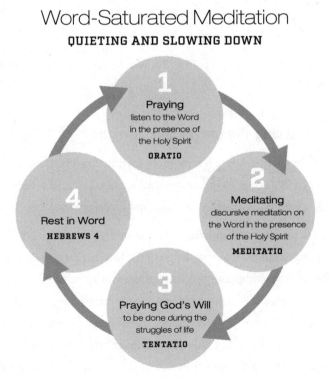

1 Praying listen to the Word in the presence of the Holy Spirit **ORATIO**

2 Meditating discursive meditation on the Word in the presence of the Holy Spirit **MEDITATIO**

3 Praying God's Will to be done during the struggles of life **TENTATIO**

4 Rest in Word **HEBREWS 4**

Choose Scripture text:

Choose a brief section of the Scriptures on which to meditate. Merely a few verses from any chapter will suffice. You may choose this randomly by just opening the Bible, or you may follow a prescribed sequence from a devotional guide or a lectionary appropriate to the season of the Church year. You may just use a single line for example:

"The Lord is my Shepherd, I shall not want..." (Psalm 23)

"The Lord takes pleasure in those who fear him, in those who hope in his steadfast love. (Psalm 147:11)

"Preserve me, O God, for in you I take refuge." (Psalm 16:1-2, 5, 8-9, 11)

"The Spirit helps us in our weakness...the Spirit intercedes for us with groaning too deep for words...if God is for us, who can be against us..." (Romans 8:26-32, 35-39)

"Cast all your anxiety on him because he cares for you." (1 Peter 5:7)

Before entering the prayer, begin with:

Quieting: Begin by taking a few moments of quieting, breathing slowly and deeply Try a five-count to breathe in, and a seven-count to breathe out. In doing this, your body quiets, your pulse and blood pressure reduce.

With a slowing and quieting of your body, you can proceed in the quieting of your mind. You may let go of the internal conversation that can often be so distracting, and therefore allow you to be meditating on the Word. Sometimes it is helpful to replace your own thoughts with a *breath prayer*, such as, "Lord (as you inhale), have mercy (as you exhale)." The use of a word or phrase like this helps to quiet both your mind and spirit, so that, like Mary of Bethany, you can sit at Jesus' feet and listen to God's Word. It is a mindful, Christ-focused quieting. I realize that for some, using terms like, "Lord, have mercy," or "Christ, have mercy," in this setting might be disruptive to them, so you can make this an individual choice. Merely breathing consciously will suffice.

By *pausing internal self-conversation,* you have the opportunity to *let go* of ingrained emotional-response habits and behaviors and instead hear the power of God's Word within you. A healing and restructured emotional-response pattern may begin, but it's now directed by the Holy Spirit. We come to God's Word quietly and unhurriedly to hear God's *whisper,* to open ourselves to the working of the Holy Spirit within our hearts, and to understand God's good will for us as beloved children.

The Prayer

1. Listening to the Word: As you are quieted, then offer a prayer inviting the Holy Spirit into your time of being in God's Word, asking that the Holy Spirit work God's Word and will within you. Theologians like Luther suggest reading the Word aloud so that it is heard not just by your heart, but also upon your ears.

2. Discursive meditation: Having quieted and received the Word of God, now you are praying in God's own words, in God's language, and doing so in the presence of the Holy Spirit. In this second phase of Word-saturated meditative prayer, we discursively meditate on God's Word. We can reflect on the entire text of the chosen passage, or even just a word or two of the Scripture for the day. One might allow several minutes for this time of reflection in the presence of the Spirit.

3. Praying God's will: Through the Spirit, God has worked the Word within us. However, we know that the forces of sin are also always present, tempting to separate us from the love of God. Therefore we begin a time of praying God's Word and will into our specific intentions, concerns, struggles, and yes, our praise, thanks, and celebrations of life. Here we ask that God's will, as expressed in our meditation on the Word, be applied to our daily faith-walk. We know that Satan, the desires of the world, and our own flesh will tempt us to try to separate us from our relationship with God.

4. Rest: We then take just a moment in Part Four to rest securely in the Word, being held in the arms of our Savior, the Good Shepherd. Being refreshed by being in God's holy Word, we may be guided back into the Scriptures for further reflection, or be released into the activities of our day.

On our Grace Place Wellness Retreats we suggest three cycles of this meditative prayer format. First, we read the Scripture text aloud and meditate on the entire chosen text for the day. In the second cycle, again reading the text aloud, we focus on just a word or phrase from the text on which to reflect silently under the guidance of the Holy Spirit. Third, because we do this in a group setting, after reading the text aloud, we take time to share our meditation aloud with each other, to receive insights from those journeying with us. Often we close the third cycle with the Lord's Prayer focused on God's will being done in our lives and for our time of personal intention.

The direction and focus is to breathe in and within the Scriptures throughout the entire prayer, including adding a moment of rest as we prepare to return to a reading of God's Word. Our intention and direction is to invite God to work the Word within us, whether actively, as the Holy Spirit guides us during the time of quiet meditation on the Word, or passively as in the time of rest, simply opening ourselves up to God to fill us with God's presence as expressed in the Word and quietly pause to dwell in God's love and light for us. God is giving; we are receiving. We eat, drink, and inwardly digest God's messages of comfort, love, peace, and joy.

Some choose to add a moment of reflective song to close your time of Word-saturated meditative prayer. For many, that can be singing a verse or two of a familiar hymn, or a Christian-based song. Here's a few texts and tunes:

My Faith Looks Up to Thee

O God, Our Help in Ages Past

Jesus, Grant That Balm and Healing

Be Still, My Soul

A Mighty Fortress Is Our God

Turn Your Eyes Upon Jesus

Breathe on Me, Breath of God

Finally, go in peace and serve the Lord throughout your day.

Here are a few additional resources:

1. Search for "Oratio, Meditatio, Tentatio" and "Martin Luther"—for example, "Oratio, Meditatio, Tentiatio: What Makes a Theologian," *Concordia Theological Quarterly* 66/3 (2002): 255-67 or www.johnkleining.com.

2. Search for topics under "contemplative outreach" and "Father Thomas Keating"—for example, www.comtemplativeoutreach.org.

3. Examine multiple texts or articles exploring Lectio Divina by St. Augusting, such as "Ever Ancient, Ever New: The Art and Practice of Lectio Divina" at www.usccb.org.

ENDNOTES

1. Manage Your Career: About how many jobs will the average person have in his or her lifetime? 2017. Experience, Inc. https://www.experience.com

2. Frost R, The Road Not Taken, *Mountain Interval, 1916.*

3. Hayes KJ. *Aging in Aspen: How long do you want to live?* Aspen Times Weekly, July 20, 2017.

4. Aubert G, Lansdorp PM, Telomeres and Aging, *Physiol Rev* 88:557-579, 2008.

5. Hassing RF, Descartes on God, Creation, and Conservation, *The Review of Metaphysics* 64 (March 2011): 603-620.

6. Iglesias, T, *What Does it Mean to be Human?* Adapted from Theresa Iglesias, *The Dignity of the Individual: Issues of Bioethics and Law.* Pleroma Press, Dublin, 2001. pp 69-72.

7. Kolb, Robert. Personal communication, November, 2017.

8. "Temperature Regulation of the Human Body." Hyperphysics.py-astr.gsu.edu. Retrieved 2017-03-01.

9. Jelkmann W (2007)"Erythropoietin after a century of research: younger than ever." *European Journal of Haematology.* 78 (3): 183-205.

10. Buettner, Dan, *Blue Zones: The Science of Living Longer: 9 Lessons for Living Longer from the People Who've Lived the Longest,* National Geographic Partners, LLC, 2008, 2012.

11. National Geographic Partners, LLC, Special Publication, Time Inc. Specials, 2016

12. Neergaard, Lauran, *New Frontier in cancer care: Turning blood into living drugs,* Aspen Daily News, AP Medical Press, June 13, 2017.

13. Taashi Makinodan, and Edmond Yunis, Eds. *Immunology and Aging,* Plenum Medical Book Company, New York and London, 1977.

14. Massoud, Ahmad and Rszaei, Nima, Eds. *Immunology of Aging.* Springer, 2014.

15. Aspinall R, Del Giudice G, Effros RB, Grubeck-Loebenstein G, Saubharas S. Challenges for vaccination in the elderly. *Immun Ageing.* 2007;4:9.

16. Monto AS, Amsaldi F, Aspinall R, et al. Influenza control in the 21st century: optimizing protection of older adults. *Vaccine.* 2009;27(37):5043-5053.

17. Lal H, et al. Efficiency of an Adjuvanted Herpes Zoster Subunit Vaccine in Older Adults. *N Engl J of Med.* 2015;372:2087-96.

18. Austrian R, Douglas RM, Schiffman G, et al (1976). "Prevention of pneumococcal pneumonia by vaccination." *Tran Assoc Am Physicians.* 89: 184-94. PMID 14433.

19. Aiello, A, Acardi, G, et al, 2016. Nutrigerontology: A Key for Achieving Successful Aging and Longevity. *Immunity and Ageing,* 13(1), 17.

20. Garia AMC, Gomes-Santos AC, Goncalves JL, Moreira TG, Medeiros SR, Dourado LPA, and Cara DC, 2013. Food Components and the Immune System: From Tonic Agents to Allergens. *Frontiers in Immunology,* 4.

21. Linus Pauling Institutes. "Macronutrient Information Center." Oregon State University, Accessed March 19, 2012 from https://lpi.oregonstate.edu/inforcenter/phytochemicals/resveratrol.

22. Environmental Nutrition, Volume 41 Issue 1, January 2018; www.environmentalnutrition.com/cs.

23. Durnas C, Loi CM, Cusack BJ. Hepatic drug metabolism and aging. *Clin Pharmacokinet.* 1990.

24. Heidelbaugh JJ, 2013. Proton Pump Inhibitors and Risk of Vitamin and Mineral Deficiency: Evidence and Clinical Implications. *Theraputic Advances in Drug Safety,* 4(3), 125-133

25. Filion K, 2016. Proton Pump Inhibitors and Community Acquired Pneumonia, *BMJ,* 2016;355:i6041.

26. Noth RH, Mazzaferri EL, Age and the endocrine system, *Clin Geriatr Med.* 1985 Feb; 1(1):223-50.

27. Noth RH, Mazzaferri EL, Age and the endocrine system, *Clin Geriatr Med.* 1985 Feb; 1(1):223-50.

28. Selmer C, Oelsen JB, Hansen ML, et al. Subclinical and overt thyroid dysfunction and risk of all-cause mortality and cardiovascular events: a large population study. *J Clin Endocrinol Metab.* 2014;99 (7):2372-2382. PMID: 24654753 www.ncbi.nlh.nih.gov/pubmed/24654753.

29. Skaznik-Wikiel ME, Traub ML, Santoro N. Menopause. In: Jameson JL, De Groot LJ, de Kretzer DM, et al, eds. *Endocrinology: Adult and Pediatric.* 7th ed. Philadelphia, PA: Elsevier Saunders; 2016;chap 135.

30. Wikipedia. Cell Death and Differentiation.

31. Baynes JW. Aging. In: Baynes JW, Dominiczak MH, eds. *Medical Biochemistry.* 4th ed. Philadelphia, PA: Elsevier Saunders; 2014:chap 43.

32. Walston JD. Common sequelae of aging. In: Goldman L, Schafer AL. eds. *Goldman-Cecil Medicine.* 25th ed. Philadelphia, PA: Elsevier Saunders; 2016:chap 25.

33. Masoro EJ. The physiology of aging. In: Boron WF, Boulpaep EL, eds. *Medical Physiology.* Updated 2nd ed. Philadelphia, PA: Elsevier Saunders; 2012:chap 62.

34. Walston JD. Common sequelae of aging. In: Goldman L, Schafer AL. eds. *Goldman-Cecil Medicine.* 25th ed. Philadelphia, PA: Elsevier Saunders; 2016:chap 25.

35. Donofrio LM. Evaluation and management of the aging face. In: Robinson JK, Hanke CW, Siegel DM, Fratila A, Bhatia AC, Rohrer TE, eds. *Surgery of the Skin.* 3rd ed. Philadelphia, PA: Elsevier Saunders; 2015:chap 23.

36. Brodie SE, Francia JH. Aging and disorders of the eye. In: Fillit HM, Rockwood K, Young J. eds. *Brocklehurst's Textbook of Geriatric Medicine and Gerontology.* 8th ed. Philadelphia, PA: Elsevier Saunders; 2017:chap 95.

37. Minaker KL. Common clinical sequelae of aging. In Goldman L, Schafer Al. eds. *Goldman-Cecil Medicine.* 24th ed. Philadelphia, PA: Elsevier Saunders; 2011:chap 24.

38. Aronson JK. Sunscreens. In: Aronson JK, ed. *Myler's Side Effects of Drugs.* 16 ed. Waltham, MA: Elsevier; 2016:603-604.

39. Bouchez C, Worried that your skin looks older than you feel? Here are 23 ways to reduce wrinkles-starting now! *Web*MD

40. Lamberts SWJ, van den Beld AW. Endocrinology and aging. In: Melmed S, Plonsky KS, Larsen PR, Kroneberg HM. eds. *Williams Textbook of Endocrinology.* 13th ed. Philadelphia, PA: Elsevier; 2016:chap 27.

41. Walston JD. Common sequelae of aging. In: Goldman L, Schafer AL. eds. *Goldman-Cecil Medicine.* 25th ed. Philadelphia, PA: Elsevier Saunders; 2016:chap 25.

42. Snyder PJ, Bhasin S, Cunningham GR, Matsumoto AM, Stephen-Shields Aj, Cauley JA, Gill TM, Barrett-Connor E, Swerdloff RS, Wang C, and Ensrud KE, 2016. Effects of Testosterone Treatment in Older Men. *New England Journal of Medicine,* 374(7), 611-624.

43. Walston JD. Common sequelae of aging. In: Goldman L, Schafer AL. eds. *Goldman-Cecil Medicine.* 25th ed. Philadelphia, PA: Elsevier Saunders; 2016:chap 25.

44. Smith PP, Kuche GA. Aging of the urinary tract. In: Fillit HM, Rockwood K, Young J, eds. *Brocklehurst's Textbook of Geriatric Medicine and Gerontology.* 8th ed. Philadelphia, PA: Elsevier; 2017:chap 22.

45. Griebling TL. Aging and geriatric urology. In: Wein AJ, Kavoussi LR, Partin AW, Peters CA, eds. *Campbell-Walsh Urology.* 8th ed. Philadelphia, PA: Elsevier, 2016:chap 88.

46. Urologix.com. Learn about BPH (Enlarged Prostate) Video and questionnaire.

47. Lamberts SWJ, van den Beld AW. Endocrinology and aging. In: Melmed S, Plonsky KS, Larsen PR, Kroneberg HM. eds. *Williams Textbook of Endocrinology.* 13th ed. Philadelphia, PA: Elsevier; 2016:chap 27.

48. Grady D, Barrett-Connor E. Menopause. In: Goldman L, Schafer Al, eds. *Goldman-Cecil Medicine.* 25th ed. Philadelphia, PA: Elsevier Saunders; 2016:chap 240.

49. Lobo RA. Menopause and care of the mature woman: endocrinology, consequences of estrogen deficiency, effects of hormonal therapy, and other treatment options. In: Lobo RA, Gershenson DM, Lentz GM, Valea FA, eds. *Comprehensive Gynecology.* 7th ed. Philadelphia, PA: Elsevier; 2017:chap 14.

50. Pinkerton JV, et al. The 2017 hormone therapy position statement of the North American Menopause Society. *Menopause.* 2017 Jul;24(7):728-753.

51. Walston JD. Common sequelae of aging. In: Goldman L, Schafer AL. eds. *Goldman-Cecil Medicine.* 25th ed. Philadelphia, PA: Elsevier Saunders; 2016:chap 25.

52. Davidson NE. Breast cancer and benign breast disorders. In: *Goldman-Cecil*

53. Walter LC, Schonber MA. Screening Mammography in Older Women: A Review, *JAMA,* 2014 Apr 2;311(13):1336-1347.

54. Gregson CL, Bone and joint aging. In. Fillit HM, Rockwood K, Young J. eds. *Brocklehurst's Textbook of Geriatric Medicine and Gerontology.* 8th ed. Philadelphia, PA: Elsevier; 2017:chap 20.

55. Weber TJ. Osteoporosis. In: Goldman L, Schafer Al, eds. *Goldman-Cecil Medicine.* 25th ed. Philadelphia, PA: Elsevier Saunders; 2916:chap 25.

56. Institute of Medicine, Food and Nutrition Board. Dietary Reference Intakes for Calcium and Vitamin D. National Academy Press, Washington, D.C. 2011. PMID:21796828 www.ncbi.nih.gov/pubmed/21796828.

57. Kling JM, Clare BL, Sandhu NP. Osteoporosis Prevention, Screening, and Treatment: A Review. *J Women's Health Treatment* (Larchmt). 2014 Jul 1;23(7):563-572.

58. Nikhra V. (2017, September 18). Aging Heart: Recent Research and Concepts. Retrieved from http://crimsonpublishers.com/ggs/pdf/GGS.000501.pdf.

59. Lanier JB, Mote MB, and Clay EC, 2011. Evaluation and management of orthostatic hypotension. *American Family Physician,*

60. Stone NJ, Robinson JG, Lichtenstein AH, et al. 2013 ACC/
    AHA guideline on the treatment of blood cholesterol to reduce
    atherosclerotic cardiovascular risk in adults: a report of the
    American College of Cardiology/American Heart Association
    Task Force on Practical Guidelines. *Circulation.* 2014: 129 (25
    Suppl 2): S1-S45. PMID:24222016 www.ncbi.nlm.nih.gov/
    pubmed;24222016

61. Tedesco S, Baron J, and O'Flynn B, 2017. A Review of Activity
    Trackers for Senior Citizens: Research Perspectives, Commercial
    Landscape and the Role of the Insurance Industry. *Sensors,* 17(6),
    p. 1277, and, Kloot GS, 2017. The Effects of Aging on Lung
    Structure and Function. *Clinics in Geriatric Medicine,* 33(4),
    pp.447-457.

62. Walston JD. Common sequelae of aging. In: Goldman L, Schafer
    AL. eds. *Goldman-Cecil Medicine.* 25th ed. Philadelphia, PA:
    Elsevier Saunders; 2016:chap 25.

63. Amin P, Smith AM. Pulmonary disease. In: Hamm RJ, Sloane
    PD, Warshaw GA, Potter JF, Flaherty E, eds. *Primary Care
    Geriatrics:* A Case-Based Approach. 6th ed. Philadelphia, PA:
    Elsevier Saunders; 2014:chap 48.

64. Davies Ga, Bolton DE. Age-related changes in the respiratory
    system. In: Fillit HM, Rockwood K, Young J, eds. *Brocklehurst's
    Textbook of Geriatric Medicine and Gerontology.* 8th ed.
    Philadelphia, PA: Elsevier; 2017:chap 17.

65. Skloot GS, 2017. The Effects of Aging on Lung Structure and
    function. *Clinics in Geriatric Medicine,* 33(4), 447-457.

66. Le Cann P, Paulus H, Glorennec P, Le Bot, F, Frain S, and
    Gangneuz JP, 2017, Home Environmental Interventions for
    the Prevention or Control of Allergic and Respiratory Diseases:

What Really Works. *The Journal of Allergy and Clinical Immunology: In Practice,* 5(1), 66-79.

67. Walston JD. Common sequelae of aging. In: Goldman L, Schafer AL. eds. *Goldman-Cecil Medicine.* 25th ed. Philadelphia, PA: Elsevier Saunders; 2016:chap 25.

68. Bubu OM, Brannick M, Mortimer J, Umasabor-Bubu O, Sebastiao YV, Wen Y, Schwartz S, Borenstein AR, Wu Y, Morgan D, and Anderson WM, 2017, Sleep, Cognitive Impairment and Alzheimer's Disease: A Systematic Review and Meta-Analysis. *Sleep,* 40(1).

69. Osorio RS, Pirraglia E [...]Leon MJ, Greater Risk of Alzheimer's Disease in Older Adults with Insomnia, *Journal of the American Geriatrics Society.* 2011 Mar; 59(3): 559-562.

70. Sterniczuk R, Rusak B. Sleep in relation to aging, frailty, and cognition. In. Fillit HM, Rockwood K, Young J, eds. *Brocklehurst's Textbook of Geriatric Medicine and Gerontology.* 8th ed. Philadelphia, PA; Elsevier; 2017:chap 108.

71. Galvin JE. Neurologic signs in older adults. In: Fillit HM, Rockwood K, Young J, eds. *Brocklehurst's Textbook of Geriatric Medicine and Gerontology,* 8th ed. Philadelphia, PA: Elsevier; 2017:chap 18.

72. Khandelwal C, Kaufr Dl. Alzheimer's disease and other dementias. In: Ham RJ, Sloane PD, Warshaw GA, Potter JF, Flaherty E, eds. *Ham's Primary Care Geriatrics.* 6th ed. Philadelphia, PA: Elsevier Saunders; 2014:chap 17.

73. Khan BA, Boustani MA. Delerium. In: Ham RJ, Sloane PD, Warshaw GA, Potter JF, Flaherty E, eds. *Ham's Primary Care Geriatrics.* 6th ed. Philadelphia, PA: Elsevier Saunders; 2014:chap 16.

74. Albert MS, James K, Savage CR, Beckman L, Seeman T, Blazer D. Predictors of cognitive change in older persons: MacArthur studies of successful aging. Psychol Aging 1995: 10:578-589.

75. Blanchard-Fields F, Chen Y. Adaptive cognition and aging. Am Behav Scientist 1996; 39:231-248.

76. Horn JL, Cattell RB. Age differences in fluid and crystallized intelligence. Acta Psychol 1967; 26:107-129.

77. Lowsky DJ, Olhansky SJ, Bhattacharya J, Goldman DP. Heterogeneity in Healthy Aging. *The Journals of Gerontology: Series A,* Issue 6, June 1, 2013, ppss. 640-649.

78. Kaufman AS, Reynolds CR, McLean JE. Age and WAIS-R intelligence in a national sample of adults in the 20 to 4-year range: a cross-sectional analysis with educational level controlled. Intelligence 1989; 13:235-253.

79. Lezak MD. The normal cognitive aging of older personas. Neuropsychological assessment. New York: Oxford University Press; 1995, pp 288-296; and, Lovelace EA. Cognitive aging: a summary overview. In: Lovelace EA, ed. Aging and cognition: mental processes, self-awareness and intervention. Amsterdam (North-Holland): Elsevier Science Publishers; 1990, pp 407-434.

80. Farmer ME, Kittner SJ, Rae DS, Barto JJ, Regier DA. Education and change in cognitive function: The Epidemiologic Catchment Area Study. Ann Epidemiol 1995; 5:1-7.

81. Smith PJ, Blumenthal JA, Sherwood A. Aerobic Exercise and Neurocognitive Performance: A Meta-Analytic Review of Randomized Controlled Trials. *Psychosomatic Medicine. 2010 April; 72(3): 239-252; and* Baumgart M, Snyder HM, Carrillo MC, Fazio S, Kim H, Johns H. Summary of the evidence on modifiable risk factors for cognitive decline and dementia: a population-based perspective. *Alzheimer's & Dementia,*

published on line: May 31, 2015. https://doi.org/*10.1016/j.jalz2015.05.016.*

82. Kang H, Zhao F, You L, Giorgetta C, Venkatesh D, Sarkhel S, Prakash R. Pseudo-dementia: A neuropsychological review, *Annals of Indian Academy of Neurology.* 2014 Apr-Jn; 17(2: 147-154.

83. Entis L. Brain Games Don't Work. Fortune. http://fortune.com/2017/07/10/brain-games-research-lumosity/. Published July 10, 2017. Accessed January 8, 2018.

84. Shah, Tejal M., et al. "Enhancing cognitive functioning in healthy older adults: a systematic review of the clinical significance of commercially available computerized cognitive training in preventing cognitive decline." Neuropsychology review 27.1 (2017): 62-80.

85. Hayslip B, Maloy RM, Kohl R. Long-term efficacy of fluid ability interventions with older adults. J Gerontol Soc Sci 1995; 50B: pp 141-149.

86. Stigsdotter-Neely A, Backman L. Effects of multifactorial memory training in old age: generalizability across tasks and individuals. J Gerontol Soc Sci: 995; 50B: pp 134-140.

87. Bamidis PD, Vivas AB, Styliadis C, Frantzidi C, A Review of Physical and Cognitive Interventions in Aging; *Elsevier,* Volume 44, July 2014, PP 206-220.

88. Rice MM, Graves AB, McCurry SM, Larson EB. Estrogen replacement therapy and cognitive function in post-menopausal women without dementia. Am J Med 1997; in press.

89. Sherwin BB. Estrogen effects on cognition in menopausal women. Neurology 1997; 48 (Suppl 7): 521-526

90. Teri L, McCurry SM, Logsdon RG. Memory, thinking, and aging. What we know about what we know. West J Med. 1997, Oct; 167(4): 269-275.

91. Geldmacher DS, Whitehouse PJ. Differential diagnosis of Alzheimer's disease. Neurology 1997: 48 (Suppl 6): 52-59.

92. Schellenberg GD, Bird JD, Wijsman EM, Orr HT, Anderson L, Nemens E, et al. Genetic linkage evidence for a familial Alzheimer's disease locus on chromosome. Science 1992: 258:668-671.

93. Traber MG, Sies H. Vitamin E in humans: demand and delivery. Ann Rev Nutri 1996: 16: 321-347.

94. Lancaster E. The Diagnosis and Treatment of Autoimmune Encephalitis. *Journal of Clinical Neurology (Seoul, Korea).* 2016;12(1):1-13. doi:10.3988/jcn.2016.12.1.1.

95. Samo M, Ernesto C, Thomas RG, Klauber MR, Schafer K, Grundman M, et al. A controlled trial of selegiline alpha-tocopherol, or both as treatment for Alzheimer's disease. N Engl J Med 1997; 336:1216-1222.

96. Alzheimer's disease." International journal of geriatric psychiatry 23.11 (2008): 1156-1162.

97. Frith, Emily, and Paul D. Loprinzi. "Physical activity is associated with higher cognitive function among adults at risk for Alzheimer's disease." Complementary Therapies in Medicine 36 (2018): 46-49.

98. Ownby, Raymond L., et al. "Depression and risk for Alzheimer disease: systematic review, meta-analysis, and meta-regression analysis." Archives of general psychiatry 63.5 (2006): 530-538.

99. Saczynski, Jane S., et al. "The effect of social engagement on incident dementia: the Honolulu-Asia Aging Study." American Journal of Epidemiology 163.5 (2006): 433-440.

100. Scarmeas, Nikolaos, et al. "Physical activity, diet, and risk of Alzheimer disease." Jama 302.6 (2009): 627-637.

101. Sen, Chetana, and Krishnarpan Chatterjee. "Mid-life modifiable risk factors for late life Alzheimer's disease." Annals of Indian Academy of Neurology 17.1 (2014): 138.

102. Ratner E, and Atkinson D, 2015. Why Cognitive Training and Brain Games Will Not Prevent or Forestall Dementia. *Journal of the American Geriatrics Society, 63(12), 2612-2614.*

103. Ruthirakuhan M, Luedke AC, Tam A, Goel A, Kurji A, and Garcia A, 2012. Use of Physical and Intellectual Activities and Socialization in the Management of Cognitive Decline of Aging and in Dementia: A Review. *Journal of Aging Research,* 2012.

104. Pillai JA, and Verghese J, 2009. Social Networks and Their Role in Preventing Dementia. *Indian Journal of Psychiatry,* 51(Suppl 1), S22.

105. Small G, Vorgan G. *2 Weeks To A Younger Brain.* Boca Rotan, FL: Humanix Books, 2016.

106. Small G, Vorgan G. *The Alzheimer's Prevention Program: Keep Your Brain Healthy for the Rest of Your Life.* New York, NY: Workman Publishing Company, 2012.

107. Eckrich JD, *Fear, Anxiety and Wellness: Journey to a Heart at Peace,* Tenth Power Publishing, 2016. Chap 5.

108. Doyle, A, *How Often Do People Change Jobs,* thebalance.com. (updated May 01, 2017).

109. Bhagwa-gita, Chapter 13: Verses 8-12, Nature, the Enjoyer, and Consciousness

110. Ren, Confucianism, Wikipedia.

111. Do-Dinh Pierre. *Confucius and Chinese Humanism.* Funk & Wagnalls, New York. 1969

112. Slider, Ab, *Egyptian heart and soul conception (http://enc.slider. com/Enc/Ab_(Egyptian_heart-soul_concept))*

113. *Oxford Guide: The Essential Guide to Egyptian Mythology,* James P. Allen, p. 28, Berkley, 2003, ISBN 0-425-19096-X.

114. Frankfort, Henri (2011). *Ancient Egyptian Religion: An Interpretation.* Courier Corporation. P. 100. ISBN 978-0-486-431138-5.

115. Jones, David (2009) *the Gift of Logos: Essays in Continental Philosophy,* Cambridge Scholars Publishing. Pp33-35.

116. Aristotle. *On the Soul;* Book III, Chapter 5, pp.430a24-5.

117. Cornford FM, *Greek Religious Thought, p.64, referring to Pindar, Fragment 131.*

118. Johnston, Mark (6 July 2009), "6", *Saving God,* Princeton: Princeton University Press, p. 88, 2012-11-17.

119. Matt, Jenson (2006). *Gravity of Sin.* T & T Clark. 2012-11-17.

120. Walker DP, *The Decline of Hell: Seventeenth-Century Discussions of Eternal Torment,* 1964, p 35.

121. Michelet J, trans. William Hazlett, Letter to Nicholas Amsdorf, January 13, 1522, *The Life of Luther,* 1862, p 133.

122. Althaus, P, *The Theology of Martin Luther.* Fortress Press: Philadelphia, PA, 1966.

123. Kolb R, The Reformation of Dying and Burial: Preaching, Pastoral Care, and Ritual at Committal in Luther's Reform,

Concordia Theological Quarterly, Concordia Theological Seminary, 2017.

124. UCG.org/Bible Study Tools/Booklets/Heaven and Hell What Does the Bible Really Teach? January 24, 2011, United Church of God.

125. Bible.knowing-jesus.com/topics/Sleep-and-Death

126. Hiebert D. Edmond, *the Thessalonian Epistles,* Moody, Chicago, IL. 1971. pp 188-189.

127. Jackson, W. "Are the Dead "Asleep"?" *Christian'Courier.com* https://www.christiancourier.com/articles/663-are-the-dead-asleep

128. Kolb R, The Reformation of Dying and Burial: Preaching, Pastoral Care, and Ritual Committal in Luther's Reform, *Concordia Theological Quarterly,* January/April, 2017, *pp.* 77-94.

129. Evener V, Wittenberg's Wandering Spirits: Discipline and the Dead in the Reformation, *Church History,* Cambridge University Press, Vol.84, Issue 3, September 2015, pp.531-555.

130. Dingle I, ed., Die Bekenntnisschriten der Evangelischen-Lutherischen Kirche: Vollstandige Neuedition *(Gottingen: Vandenhoeck & Rupricht,* 2014), 734-735, lines 13-18.

131. Kolb R and Wengert T, eds., *The Book of Concord* (Minneapolis: Fortress, 2000), 304 (=SA II II 16-17).

132. Gibbs J, personal communication, Dec. 4, 2017.

133. Brighton l, *Concordia Commentary: Revelations,* Concordia Publishing House, St. Louis, 1999.

134. Schouppe FX, (2010). *Abridged course of religious instruction, apologetic, dogmatic, and moral: for the use of Catholic colleges and schools.* Burns & Oates. P. 248.

135. Kolb R, Personal Communication, December, 2017.

136. Oxford-English Dictionary (online full edition, *Soul (noun)*, December 2016.

137. Evans, Rachel Held, *Aristotle vs. Jesus: What Makes the New Testament Household Codes Different,* rachelheldevans.com, August 28, 2013.

138. "soul." Encyclopaedia Britannica. 2010. Encyclopaedia Britannica 006 CD. 13 July 2010.

139. Barber J, (2008). The Road from Eden: Studies in Christianity and Culture. *Academica Press,* p. 233.

140. "Catechetische Schriften: (1542), in *Schriften,* vol. 11, pp 287, 288.

141. "Auslegung des ersten Buches Mose" (1544), in *Schriften,* vol. 1, col.1756; and "Kirchen-Postille" (1528), in *Schriften,* vol. 11, col. 1143, *Schriften,* vol. 2, col.1069; and *Deutsche Schriften* (Erlangen ed.), vol. 11, p. 142ff; vol. 41 (1525), p. 373.

142. Froom, LE, *Conditionalist Faith of our Fathers,* Vol II, Chapter 4.

143. Kolb, Robert, personal communication, September 2017.

144. Luther, Martin. *Large Catechism,* Concordia Publishing House, (2010). Original publish date from Luther 1529.

145. Erikson E, Insight and Responsibility (New York: Norton, 1964) 81-107; Identity, Youth and Crisis (New York: Norton, 1968), 91-141; Life History and the Historical Movement (New York Norton, 1975).

146. Arand C, Two Kinds of Righteousness as a Framework for Law and Gospel in the Apology, *Lutheran Quarterly XV* (2001): 420-421.

OTHER BOOKS BY JOHN D. ECKRICH, M.D.

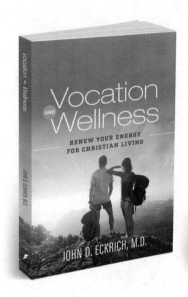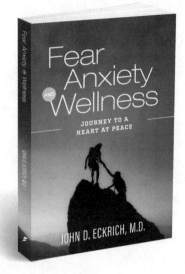

Vocation and Wellness:
Renew Your Energy for Christian Living

Fear, Anxiety, and Wellness:
Journey to a Heart at Peace

Available in print and e-book formats at online retailers.

Visit www.graceplacewellness.org for more information.